HeartMath Brain Fitness Program

*Connecting Heart and Mind
for Optimal Performance*

Deborah Rozman, Ph.D.
&
Rollin McCraty, Ph.D.

HeartMath Brain Fitness Program

Connecting Heart and Mind for Optimal Performance

Foreword
By
Daniel Amen, M.D.

Fall in Love with Your Brain and Your Heart

For the last twenty-five years I have been helping people optimize the physical functioning and working patterns of their brain. I have conducted over 85,000 brain scans and worked with tens of thousands of people.

The deep limbic system of the brain helps set our emotional tone. The emotional shading of the limbic system is the filter through which we interpret events of the day. The more positive experiences we have, the more positive we are likely to feel and to perceive events that happen in life from a more balanced perspective.

I have spent many years studying the deep limbic system and it was new information for me to learn that the core cells of the amygdala synchronize to the heart beat. The amygdala literally marches to the beat of the heart's drumming. What HeartMath discovered is that we can better self-regulate our emotions by learning how to self-regulate our heart rhythms. That sayings like, "put your heart into it" and "listen to your heart" really do affect our perceptions and moods, our sense of meaning and purpose. HeartMath has opened a new window into brain fitness by including the heart in the process.

The brain is an organ of love and now it's not just poets or our own subjective feelings telling us; now scientists are proving that the heart really is an organ of love too.

The brain is an organ of loving, learning and behavior, and so is the heart. HeartMath has demonstrated how getting the heart and brain working together can optimize mental and emotional and physical health, our sense of meaning, our relationships—our life.

The heart can help power and direct the brain. Heart coherence synchronizes brain waves and heart rhythms. It helps people build skills to enhance limbic bonds. Like my early pioneering work on the brain took a while for the medical community to understand and adopt, so the pioneering work of HeartMath is taking a while for the medical community to grasp. It's a paradigm shift. The heart is more than a blood pump; and the rhythmic patterns of the beating heart neurologically affect our brain function. It's a two way communication system.

Our physical heart contains its own independent nervous system, or "heart-brain," of approximately 40,000 neurons that can sense, feel, learn and remember. The heart-brain sends information to the big brain about how the body feels.

I help people fall in love with and take care of their brains. The HeartMath Brain Fitness Program can help you fall in love with your heart and how your heart and brain talk to each other.

Daniel Amen, M.D.

Medical Director, Amen Clinics, which has the world's largest database of functional brain scans related to behavior. New York Times bestselling author of *Change Your Brain, Change Your Life, Healing ADD, and Unleash the Power of the Female Brain*.

Costa Mesa, CA

Introduction
By
Daniel J. Siegel, M.D.

Strengthening the Mind

HeartMath provides a research-supported approach to reducing stress and improving cognitive and emotional capacities in children, adolescents and adults. This booklet offers some fascinating proposals as to how focusing on your inner physiological processes—such as the sensation of your heart beating and your breath—can produce these important improvements in how you can more effectively regulate your emotions, mood, attention and create a sense of well-being in your life. Their essential suggestion is that coordinating the rhythms of the heart with the functions of the brain enhances how the mind functions. To deeply understand the power of this notion of the interconnection between heart and brain, and between body and mind, we need to take a step back and ask the question of how these entities may be related to one another.

In the work I do in bringing the many fields of science together into one framework, a field called Interpersonal Neurobiology (IPNB), what emerges is the realization that our various academic and clinical fields focusing on the mind actually have no definition of what the mind is. For a philosopher or researcher, this presents a lifelong challenge to explore and define the mind. For the clinician or educator, this lack of a definition of mind presents a fundamental problem as a professional of how to strengthen the mind or help the mind develop well. I'll suggest to you that offering a proposal as to "what the mind is" can help us to make sense of how specific interventions, like HeartMath and other research-proven approaches to strengthening the mind, may in fact actually work.

While we know that the term, "mind" is often used to refer to our subjective experience and consciousness, and the mental activities of our thinking, feeling, remembering and decision-making, amazingly we actually don't really have a scientific explanation for what these "activities" actually are. Some suggest that they are simply outcomes of brain activity, this view stating something like "the mind is what the brain does." This is a simple suggestion that may be partly true, but it misses a number of crucial considerations such as not acknowledging the important role of the whole body beyond the skull in shaping our feelings and thoughts. Saying that the mind is simply brain activity also leaves out the whole set of dynamic interactions we have between our bodily selves and the larger world—especially within the world of our social relationships—and how these important interactions shape our mental lives. We see how the communication we have within our relationships at home, in school, in our communities and in our larger culture directly shape virtually everything that is included as what the "mind" is all about. The mind is as much relational as it is embodied. To say that the mind is simply "enskulled"—that it is simply the same as brain activity—misses so much of the reality of our mental lives.

To address these issues, IPNB looks deeply at our social and our synaptic selves, examining how our relationships and our neuronal connections, our synapses, shape the mind. In basic terms, our mind—our patterns of feelings, thoughts and behavior—is shaped by both our bodies and our relationships. But what could it be that is shared by the body and by relationships? One reasonable answer to this basic question of what body and relationships share in common is the flow of energy. For example, as you read these words, energy in the form of photons of light passes from the page to your eyes. And within your eyes, this energy of photons is converted into electrical energy as your optic nerve is activated by your retina's response to light. This neural activation is the creation of something called an "action potential"—the "firing" of the nerve—which leads to the release of neurotransmitter, a chemical, at the downstream end of the neuron where it will link to another neuron. This linkage among neurons is called a synapse, and it is the release of chemical energy in the form of neurotransmitter that either activates, or inhibits, that post-synaptic neuron's firing. In a basic way, the nervous system functions by this electrochemical energy flow, stimulated by the receiving of energy from the outside world. In fact, relationships can be defined by how we share patterns of energy between us, like from me to you right now.

Some patterns of energy have symbolic value, which means that they "stand for" something other than the energy flow itself. When this happens, we call this particular pattern of energy flow, "information." Sometimes energy patterns are in certain rhythms that are just themselves, pure energy flow, and sometimes they are symbolic, like these photons here: Golden Gate Bridge. There is no bridge, just the photons that have a shared meaning between you and me because we each share a common language.

And so we can say that relationships are the sharing of energy and information and that the body is the embodied mechanism of energy and information flow. What then is the mind? In IPNB we propose that besides subjective experience, and besides consciousness (two important aspects of mind we won't delve into more here), there is a third aspect of mind that can in fact be defined as an emergent property that arises from the complex system of energy and information flow of our lives. What is a complex system? A complex system has the three features of being chaos-capable, open and non-linear, meaning that it can become randomly distributed, is influenced by things from outside of itself, and that small inputs can lead to large and unpredictable results. Sound like your life? We are non-linear, open, chaos capable creatures—so we are in essence complex systems. When a system is complex, it has "emergent" properties, ones that arise from the coherent interactions of the system's elements across time. It appears that there is no programmer, or master controller. One relevant emergent property is that of self-organization.

Self-organization and self-regulation move a system in an ever-unfolding way by coordinating the flow of its elements across time. When those elements are able to differentiate, like left from right, or up from down in a body—or like me from you in a relationship—we see that the system achieves a level of specialization. Then when those differentiated elements become linked we say that the system is in a coherent flow that is "integrated." Integration is not blending where the components' distinctions dissolve but instead are connected through open channels of communication so that they can become coordinated and balanced. Integration is a verb, an active unfolding of a way we continually shape the linkage of differentiated parts of a system. Integration is how the whole is greater than the sum of its parts.

Integration creates the optimal self-organization and function of a system.

One word to describe the outcome of this state of integration is harmony. Think of a choir singing a song in which the individual singers can differentiate their voices in harmonic intervals while simultaneously linking together with all the others in the choir in the flow and rhythm of the song (imagine something like "Amazing Grace", for example). The feeling one gets when hearing such harmony is energizing and full of life.

The core features of integrative harmony are being flexible, adaptive, coherent, energized and stable. This overall flow of integrative harmony can be remembered as the acronym, FACES. Coherent is a mathematical term meaning how well something holds together in a fluid and dynamic way over time. This FACES flow moves along a kind of river of integration, a flow with harmony in the middle, and chaos on one bank, rigidity on the other.

So our proposal is that the mind can be defined this way: "An embodied AND relational, emergent self-organizing process that REGULATES the flow of energy and information." In brief, this aspect of mind is "an embodied and relational process that regulates the flow of energy and information."

To understand how practical this definition is, we can turn to the central part of the definition, self-regulation, and realize that to regulate something you need to do two things: monitor and modify that which you are regulating. Where does regulation take place? Within you—in your body—and between you and others—in your relationships. Within and between are the two simultaneous locations of the mind. I know this sounds unusual, but it fits with so much diverse scientific data across a range of disciplines, from physics to biology, psychology to anthropology. Wherever the mind ultimately resides, how can you strengthen or improve your mind? Making your mind stronger, enabling it to move your life toward integration and health, comes from strengthening your ability to regulate energy and information flow. Once we've defined the mind as, in part, being a regulatory process, we can see that strengthening the mind has these two fundamental steps:

Stabilizing Monitoring: When we give the gift of teaching ourselves to stabilize the lens through which we sense energy and information flow, we can see with more focus, depth, and detail. This is how we create a tripod to stabilize what I call a "mindsight lens." HeartMath stabilizes this lens by teaching you how to sense energy flow in the body (for example, thoughts and emotions) with repeated practice that builds your mindsight tripod, stabilizing your ability to see the sea inside, and seeing more clearly what is there. Many people don't have this skill of seeing inside, and this important skill can be mastered with practice.

Modulating Toward Integration: When we have stabilized our attention to the inner world and can see this sea of energy flow inside with more focus, depth, and detail, we can then modulate what we see. The way to carry out such modification of energy and information flow toward health is to move our system toward integration. My proposal to you is that linking differentiated aspects of energy and information flow—creating integration—is exactly what HeartMath is doing as it creates increased Coherence as reflected in our Heart Rate Variability in the deep physiological mechanisms underlying these basic bodily states. As we measure these objective physiological shifts, we are probably measuring states of differentiation and linkage—of integration—of the core functions of the heart, brain and the autonomic nervous system as it extends throughout the body.

The exact mechanisms at work will likely be clarified in the years and decades of research ahead, but for now the practical point that is supported by a range of scientific findings is that by focusing on the interior of the body—a process called "interoception"—we increase the function and the structural connections of important integrative areas of the brain, such as the prefrontal cortex, including an area called the insula, which can support the coordination and balance of our overall nervous system. Other studies suggest that focusing on the positive emotions of love, gratitude and joy—also fundamental steps in the HeartMath approach as they are in some contemplative practices—leads to important integrative states of brain functioning.

Taken as a whole, my suggestion to you is that we can envision how the focus of your attention toward positive emotional states and internal bodily processes like the sense of the rhythm of the heart and breath create the foundations for 1) strengthening your ability to stabilize your monitoring skills; 2) teaching you the skill of creating integration in the flow of energy and information in your body; and 3) creating a coherent, integrated state of clarity and calm that enable you to create more integration in your inner life and also extending this state of equanimity and connection into your interpersonal life.

When we place this focus of attention and modulation toward integration into awareness, we likely stabilize their states of flow in our system—as consciousness has this quality of action on our lives. Then when we practice this intentional focus of attention and the creation of integrative states and repeatedly place these in awareness on a regular basis, we are SNAGing the brain toward integration: We Stimulate Neuronal Activation and Growth to link differentiated aspects of our internal and interpersonal states. These initially effortful and intentionally created states of integration can then become more automatic as they become traits in our lives. This is how the practice of creating a coherent state grows our brains toward having the learned trait of integration in our lives.

In IPNB we see integration as the heart of health. So finding a way to make integration a trait is a natural way of building a life of well-being for yourself.

These are my "best guesses" as to why a process like HeartMath may work so well. I wish you all the best in trying the practices out for yourself. Whatever we'll discover in the future about the details of all the actual mechanisms at work, you will have now, your own experience, your own inner proof of the power of this practice. Be patient, practice and enjoy the fruits of your focus. Integrate and be well!

Daniel J. Siegel, M.D.,

Executive Director, Mindsight Institute

Author, *Brainstorm: The power and purpose of the teenage brain,*

The Developing Mind, The Mindful Brain, and Mindsight.

Los Angeles, California

About the Authors:

Deborah Rozman, Ph.D., is President and CEO of HeartMath® Inc located in Boulder Creek, California. She has been a psychologist in research and practice, and a business executive for over 30 years, and co-author with HeartMath founder Doc Childre of HeartMath's Transforming series of books (New Harbinger Publications): Transforming Anger, Transforming Stress, Transforming Anxiety and Transforming Depression. HeartMath offers scientifically validated tools, technologies and training programs that dramatically reduce stress, while empowering health, cognitive performance and behavioral change. HeartMath's award winning emWave® and Inner Balance™ technologies monitor and provide real time feedback on heart rhythm (HRV) coherence levels, an important indicator of mental and emotional state. HeartMath also offers certification programs for individuals, health professionals and organizations (www.heartmath.com).

Rollin McCraty, Ph.D., is Executive Vice President and Director of Research of the Institute of HeartMath, a research and educational organization located in Boulder Creek, California. The Institute's research has laid the foundation for the development of positive emotion-focused interventions that have been demonstrated to reduce stress, enhance health and cognitive performance, promote emotional stability, and improve quality of life (www.heartmath.org). McCraty is a Fellow of the American Institute of Stress, holds memberships with the International Neurocardiology Network, American Autonomic Society, Pavlovian Society and Association for Applied Psychophysiology and Biofeedback and is an adjunct professor at Claremont Graduate University. McCraty is an internationally recognized authority on heart-rate variability, heart-rhythm coherence and the effects of positive and negative emotions on human psychophysiology.

Table of Contents

Setting the Stage

Brain fitness is a hot topic these days and for good reason. There is a strong desire to do whatever is possible to maintain and improve our mental faculties. Cognitive decline, Alzheimer's and other mental health disorders (anxiety, depression, PTSD, etc.) are a growing concern and their costs to society will increase as the population ages. There are an increasing number of children being diagnosed with cognitive learning disabilities (especially ADHD and the autism spectrum), along with tremendous pressure on children pre-school through college to perform well on tests. There is also a concern among people of all ages about memory lapses. Even people in their 20s are reporting unusual memory lapses and difficulty focusing, while more adults in their 30s and 40s are being diagnosed with ADD/ADHD (attention deficit disorder or attention deficit hyperactivity disorder) as information overload, time pressures, too much multi-tasking and stress about the future take a toll on mental health. How often do we hear or say at the end of a stressful workday, "My brain is fried!"

In our high speed, rapidly changing society, brain fitness is becoming as important as physical and emotional fitness. In fact, they are all connected. Physical exercise, healthy diet, stress management, emotional and social well-being, and cognitive engagement provide the foundation for optimizing brain health and functions.

A foundational building block that most brain fitness programs rarely address is how our heart rhythms and emotions affect our cognitive functions—and how we can improve our minds, not only by playing puzzles and games, learning a new language or musical instrument, or going back to school, but by learning heart-based *emotional self-regulation skills*. This is what the HeartMath Brain Fitness Program provides.

Our ability to focus, concentrate and remember has a lot to do with how much emotional stress we are experiencing. Emotional stress has a major impact on our immediate and long term cognitive functions, and underlies many of the mental health problems in society today. Cognitive decline, anxiety and depression are exacerbated by the stresses and strains of modern life. It's well established by researchers that ongoing stress and worry about the future are major contributors to the decline of cognitive functions.

Neuroplasticity

Most studies show that cognitive decline starts when we are in our mid-20s. Motor skills and reaction times, an important measure of the speed of our nervous system's ability to process information, slow with age. But each of us has the ability to improve our mental functions, remain alert and develop our brain power all the way into our 80s and 90s. An exciting new discovery in the 90s was that the brain has the capacity to regenerate and grow new brain cells throughout life—a process called "neurogenesis".

More than half of people in the United States report that they have been touched by someone (living or deceased) who has Alzheimer's disease, and roughly a third of Americans are worried about getting Alzheimer's (www.alzheimersreadingroom.com). Statistics released in May 2013 from the Alzheimer's Association report that 1 in 3 American seniors die with the mind-destroying disease of Alzheimer's or another form of dementia.

ADD or ADHD (attention deficit hyperactivity disorders) affects 4–5% of adults in the USA (8 million people) and affects 3% to 10% of children in the USA. It's estimated that 60% of those children will continue to have symptoms that affect their functioning as adults.

"Neuroplasticity" has also been mentioned frequently in the news. Neuroplasticity means that the brain has the ability to change and rewire itself, to be plastic and develop new neural connections among the synapses. The brain retains this ability to change throughout the aging process. Even though our reaction times slow, we often become more thoughtful and make wiser decisions as we mature.

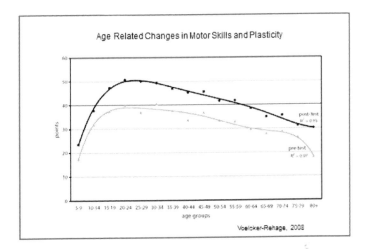

Age Related Changes in Motor Skills and Plasticity

Voelcker-Rehage, 2008

For most baby boomers, memory isn't as sharp as it once was, but other cognitive functions can be sharper than ever. Maybe now and then, we can't remember where we put the car keys or enter a room forgetting why we went there and have to retrace our steps back to where we started from to remember. But those of us who have learned emotional self-management skills and how to listen to our heart often experience our problem-solving abilities and discernment becoming more keen and refined as we age.

The good news is that it doesn't have to be one or the other. Neuroplasticity studies have shown that many brain functions which were thought to be fixed, such as working memory, are now understood to be trainable at any age. We can enhance the speed of information processes and the coordination of that information. We can sharpen our memory and become more creative and discerning. We can learn how to sustain positive emotional states and enhance our intuitive intelligence to provide us with a more positive outlook at any age.

Increasing how much time we spend in positive emotional states is a key factor in improving and sustaining cognitive functions. Experts have found that social support, volunteering in the community and learning emotional self-management can help slow down cognitive decline by increasing resilience and lowering emotional stress.

Stressful emotions that we all experience at times, like irritation, frustration, resentment, anger, worry, anxiety, fear, apathy, cause a de-synchronization in the activity of the brain and nervous system, which directly impairs cognitive functions. On the other hand, when we have a more positive outlook, when we're feeling hopeful, appreciative, caring and loving, it improves the way our brain and nervous system process information. Many older people with extraordinary cognitive capacities typically have a positive outlook, a heartfelt passion for life, and a real care about society and other people. People with these positive qualities tend to live longer and are mentally and physically healthier as they advance in age.

Heartfelt positive emotions are a tonic for the mind/brain processes. They are like a salve that smooth the transits and provide warm hearted textures that make life worth living. Who doesn't want to enjoy more love, care, compassion, kindness, and gratitude? These positive emotions are not just wonderful feelings; they are like heart oil to the brain and nervous system, creating more ease and flow through life and they give us more access to our higher brain capacities. We will discuss the physiology of how love and positive emotions affect our heart's rhythms and how these rhythms have profound effects on our mental functions in Part II.

High Cortisol /Low DHEA

Stressful emotions produce more cortisol, the stress hormone, and positive emotions are associated with more DHEA, the vitality or anti-aging hormone. Both hormones have long term effects on our cognitive functions. High cortisol can kill brain cells in the hippocampus, the brain's long term memory center, and impair learning. Long term accumulated stress and the resulting imbalances in the ratio between cortisol and DHEA are known to affect the hippocampus, as well as many other important functions involved in the aging process.

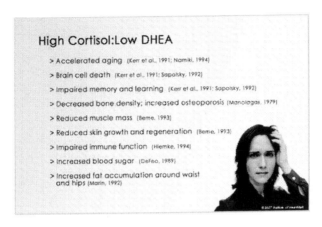

The HeartMath tools and techniques that you will use in this Brain Fitness Program have been shown to reduce cortisol and increase DHEA naturally, without the use of supplements or other dietary or lifestyle changes. The graph below shows the changes that occurred in 30 days in one study using HeartMath tools.

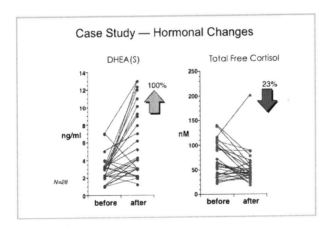

This Case Study shows how using the HeartMath tools can impact levels of both Cortisol and DHEA. In this study, 28 people practiced a HeartMath coherence building technique* for a month and saw an average 23% reduction in Cortisol and 100% increase in DHEA without changing diet or exercise. *These subjects practiced sustaining coherence for 30 minutes every day with a modified version of the Heart Lock-In® Technique. The outliers in the graph stated they did not practice.

Part I – SharpBrains

The SharpBrains Guide to Brain Fitness: How to Optimize Brain Health and Performance at Any Age (2013), by Alvaro Fernandez and Dr. Elkhonon Goldberg, selected by AARP as part of its Best Books Series, is designed to help people navigate the growing field of brain research and identify the lifestyle factors and products that contribute to brain fitness. It guides readers in the field of neuroplasticity and cognitive health. According to a report issued by SharpBrains, a market research firm, the amount spent in 2012 on brain fitness was more than a billion dollars, and by 2020, it is estimated, that figure will exceed six billion dollars. The SharpBrains Guide provides practical information for those interested in complementing other lifestyle options with a self-directed, technology-based brain fitness program.

It was to HeartMath's surprise and delight that the *SharpBrains Guide to Brain Fitness* rated our emWave® Desktop (emWave Pro) as one of the five top Brain Trainers. Out of the hundreds of products making brain training claims that SharpBrains analyzed, they found only a few that met their strict criteria indicative of high-quality and value to the user. Their first three criteria were:

1. A well-articulated scientific rationale, and at least a basic and growing level of scientific testing (Research Momentum);
2. Sustained growth among a wide variety of users (Market Momentum);
3. Higher-than-average levels of satisfaction among users with the results they have seen (Results Seen).

They developed a Brain Fitness Evaluation Checklist that asked 10 questions regarding these three criteria, including: Are there credible, university-based scientists (ideally neuropsychologists or cognitive neuroscientists) in the company's scientific advisory board? Are there peer-reviewed, scientific papers that have been published in mainstream scientific and professional journals that analyze the effects of the specific product?

SharpBrains also compiled and analyzed results from an extensive survey among subscribers of SharpBrains' monthly eNewsletter conducted in March/April of 2012, designed to elicit feedback from early-adopters and professionals in the field. Among the over 3,000 respondents, more than 1,000 identified at least one brain training product they had used (for themselves or for someone else) and answered several questions on a 5-point scale {from "strongly disagree* to "strongly agree"). A key question was whether people agreed or disagreed with the statement, "I have seen the results I wanted" and they identified the 10 companies whose products ranked highest in that question. These responses were the source for their evaluation of the third criterion, Results Seen.

SharpBrains did not endorse any of the products or technologies they analyzed, but simply pointed out the feedback from their subscribers and focus groups.

Questions they asked their focus group of users about emWave Desktop/emWave Pro and the other brain training programs that met their criteria:

1. Does the program challenge and motivate me, or does it feel like it would become easy once I learned it? (Good mental exercise requires increasing levels of difficulty and challenge.)
2. Does the program fit my personal goals? (Each individual has different goals and needs when it comes to brain health and performance. For example, some want to manage anxiety, others to improve short-term memory.)
3. Does the program fit my lifestyle? (Some programs have shown good short-term results in lab environments, but are very intense and difficult to comply with. Others may be more appropriate for more moderate use over time.)

4. Is there an independent assessment to measure my progress? (The real question is whether the improvement experienced in the program will transfer into real life.)

Out of 185 companies assessed, they found only 4 companies met all three of their criteria: Research Momentum, Market Momentum, Results Seen. HeartMath was one of those 4 companies.

SharpBrains also found EEG neurofeedback brain training devices were mostly useful as brain training tools in research and clinical contexts. In contrast, they found heart rate variability (HRV) feedback devices helped people influence their heart and brain by self-monitoring and self-regulating their breathing and emotions, and can be used by anyone, anywhere, at any time.

emWave® Technology

HeartMath's mission is to help people bring their physical, mental and emotional systems into balanced alignment with their heart's intuitive guidance, to become "who we truly are" – our full potential. We developed self-regulation and performance enhancement training programs and emWave technologies that measure heart rate variability (HRV) to show you when your heart, brain and nervous system are in balanced alignment, a state reflected by higher levels of heart rhythm coherence (see Part II). The emWave Desktop (emWave Pro) computer-based technology, the portable emWave2, and the Inner Balance™ Trainer for iOS and Android devices are front runner products for brain fitness because they facilitate learning how to shift into heart coherence and sustain heart-brain synchronization.

A key reason why emWave and Inner Balance technologies have gained such Market Momentum, Results Seen. They help clear the stress and anxiety that jams the brain when trying to focus or make decisions—while enhancing emotional balance and mental and intuitive clarity. That's why many neurofeedback practiontioners have clients first use the emWave to get their heart, brain and nervous system into alignment before neuro-feedback brain training. To know how the HeartMath Brain Fitness Program with emWave or Inner Balance technology works, it helps to understand some of the research behind it. If you want to go right to the Program and get started, you can skip the research in Part II and go to Part III.

Part II – Heart-Brain Communication

Traditionally scientists believed that the brain sent more information and issued commands to the heart, but they now know the reverse is true. The heart and brain continually exchange critical information that influences how the brain and body function. The heart actually sends far more information to the brain than the brain sends to the heart – in fact, 90 to 95% of the nerves connecting the heart and brain are afferent (ascending or going to) neural fibers carrying messages from the heart to the brain.

Researchers have also found that the heart communicates with the brain in four major ways: neurologically (through the transmission of nerve impulses); biochemically (via hormones and neurotransmitters); biophysically (through blood pressure waves); and energetically (through electromagnetic field interactions). Communication along all these pathways significantly affects the brain's activity and research shows that the messages the heart sends the brain also affects a wide range of mental functions and our performance.

In the 1960s and '70s, researchers John and Beatrice Lacey were the first to observe that the heart communicates with the brain in ways that affect how we perceive and react to the world. They found that the heart appeared to be sending meaningful messages to the brain that it not only understood, but obeyed. Even more intriguing was that it looked as though these messages could affect a person's perceptions and behavior. Shortly after this, neurophysiologists discovered the mechanisms whereby input from the heart to the brain could "inhibit" or "facilitate" the brain's activity.

The heart was reclassified as part of the hormonal system in 1983, when a new hormone produced by the heart was discovered called atrial natriuretic peptide (ANP), or atrial peptide. Nicknamed the "balance hormone," it exerts its effects on the blood vessels, kidneys, adrenal glands and many of the regulatory regions of the brain. In addition, ANP inhibits the release of stress hormones and experiments suggest that atrial peptide can influence motivation and behavior. More recently, it was discovered that the heart also produces significant amounts of the hormone called oxytocin, which has a strong influence on emotional and social behaviors.

The heart's ever-present rhythmic electromagnetic field has a powerful influence on communicative processes throughout the body. This heart's electrical voltage is about 60 times greater in amplitude than the electrical activity produced by the brain and permeates every cell in the body. Thus, the heartbeat can be detected by placing electrodes anywhere on the body, from the little toe to the top of the head. The magnetic component of the heart's field is approximately 100 times stronger than the magnetic field produced by the brain.

One of the early pioneers of this fairly new field of neurocardiology, Dr. J. Andrew Armour, published in scientific circles in 1991 that the heart contains its own complex intrinsic nervous system that is sufficiently sophisticated to qualify as a "little brain" in its own right. This heart-brain is an intricate network of several types of neurons, neurotransmitters, proteins and support cells like those found in the cranial brain. Its elaborate circuitry enables this heart-brain to act independently of the cranial brain *and to learn, remember, and even feel and sense*. The heart-brain contains around 40,000 neurons, called sensory neurites. These neurons in the heart have been shown to have both short and long term memory, just like the neurons in the hippocampus. Heart neurons also have plasticity and can change and rewire like neurons in the brain.

It's the interaction between the brain in the head and the little brain in the heart that impacts how well we function mentally. Information is sent from the heart-brain to the head brain through several afferent (flowing to the brain) neural pathways. These ascending nerve pathways enter the brain in an area called the medulla, located at the bottom of the brain. The heart's signals then cascade up into all of the higher centers of the brain, where they influence perception, decision making and other cognitive processes. Think of the heart's rhythm (the time between each and every heartbeat) as a "morse code" which contains instructions for the brain. The neural signals the heart sends to the brain are continuously monitored by the brain and they help organize our perceptions, feelings and behavior. Thus the heart directly impacts the way the brain perceives and processes information.

Of particular significance is the influence of the heart's input on the activity of our cortex—that part of the brain that governs our thinking and reasoning capacities. Depending on the nature of the heart's input, it can either *inhibit or facilitate* attention, working memory, cortical processes, mental functions and performance.

In 1993, the Institute of HeartMath (IHM) began exploring the physiological mechanisms by which the heart communicates with the brain, thereby influencing intentional focus, information processing, perceptions, emotions and health. IHM explored how the heart is, in fact, a highly complex, self-organized information encoding and processing center whose influences profoundly affect brain function and most of the body's major organs, and ultimately determine the quality of life. The heart is the most powerful generator of rhythmic information patterns in the human body. With every beat, the heart not only pumps blood, but also transmits complex patterns of neurological, hormonal, pressure and electromagnetic information to the brain and throughout the body. IHM's studies built upon research showing that: Though the heart and brain are in constant communication with each other, each of us has the capacity to consciously and intentionally direct our heart to communicate with our brain in ways that enhance our cognitive functions and our health.

Heart Coherence

IHM discovered a distinct mode of harmonious physical and psychological functioning that promotes emotional stability and optimal cognitive performance, called psycho-physiological coherence or simply "heart coherence." It's a state where heart-brain interactions, mind, emotions and nervous system are operating in sync and in energetic cooperation. Synchronized electrical activity in the brain and nervous system underlies our ability to perceive, feel, focus, learn, reason and perform at our best. Researchers found that synchronized activity can be more important than how much activity there is in our brain wave frequencies (alpha waves, beta waves, etc.) for optimal performance. It only takes a little disruption of synchronized activity to negatively affect our ability to focus, think clearly and perform at our best.

Heart coherence appears when the heart's beat-to-beat rhythm is producing a sine-wavelike pattern. When we experience sincere positive emotions, such as caring, compassion, love, appreciation, kindness for someone or something, the heart rhythm pattern becomes coherent and communicates this more harmonious pattern to the brain and entire body. During heart rhythm coherence, there can also be an increase in beat-to-beat variability in our heart rate (HRV) which results in an increase in the neural signals sent from the heart to the brain. People with higher HRV also tend to do better on cognitive function tests.

Based on this research, HeartMath created tools and programs to help us learn how to intentionally shift into a heart coherent state, and after a short time of practice, achieve a new internal baseline that improves our reaction times and many other cognitive functions. This is often experienced as an increased ability to focus, heightened mental clarity, improved decision making and increased intuition and creativity.

Emotion and Cognition

There is a strong relationship between emotion and cognition. When we experience stress and negative emotions such as anger, frustration, worry or anxiety, the heart rhythm pattern becomes erratic and disordered — creating an incoherent waveform (see top pattern on the graph on page 16). This is indicative of inhibited executive functions in our higher brain centers. The generation of this erratic pattern of heart and nervous system activity impedes the efficient flow of information throughout our nervous system and interferes with our brain's ability to properly synchronize neural activity through the entire brain. This de-synchronization impedes brain processes necessary for focused attention, memory recall, abstract reasoning, problem-solving and creativity. High levels of anxiety, frustration or anger, and the "inner noise" produced by incoherence, impairs the very cognitive resources we need for brain fitness.

On the other hand, when our heart transmits a coherent wave to the higher brain centers (see bottom pattern on graph below), we typically experience more emotional stability and enhanced attention, memory recall, comprehension, reasoning ability, intuition, creativity and task performance. *This is a particularly important point in understanding the operative mechanism of the emWave and Inner Balance technologies for brain fitness.*

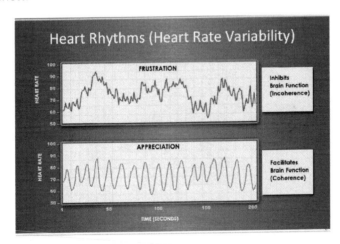

As mentioned earlier, positive emotions such as appreciation, care, compassion and love generate a smooth, sine-wave-like (coherent) pattern in the heart's rhythms. When our heart rhythm pattern is coherent, we not only feel better, the neural information sent to our brain facilitates cortical function. *With regular practice in maintaining heart coherence utilizing*

emWave or Inner Balance heart rhythm coherence feedback technology, a new coherent baseline pattern can be established that optimizes cognitive functions.

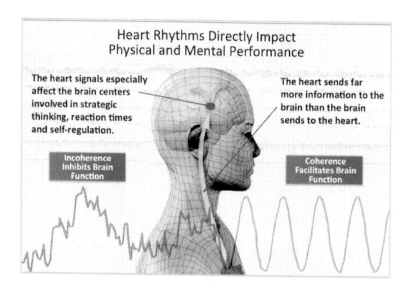

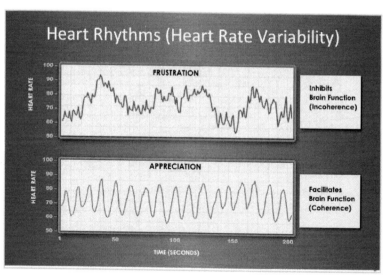

When heart coherence is generated by a positive emotional state (not just through paced breathing), it is called *psycho-physiological coherence*. This state is associated with sustained positive feeling and a high degree of mental and emotional stability. There is increased synchronization and balance between our cognitive, emotional and physiological systems, resulting in efficient and harmonious functioning of our whole being. Observed outcomes include: reduced stress, anxiety and depression; increased feelings of well-being; enhanced immunity and hormonal balance; increased ability to focus and sustain focus; improved cognitive performance and enhanced learning; increased organizational effectiveness; and physical and mental health improvements.

It's worth noting that the term "coherence" has several definitions, all of which apply when we are in psycho-physiological coherence:

Definitions of Coherence:

- The quality of being orderly, consistent and intelligible (e.g. a coherent argument)
- Clarity of thought and emotional balance
- A constructive waveform produced by two or more waves that are phase- or frequency locked (e.g. lasers)
- An ordered or constructive distribution of energy within a single waveform (e.g. sine wave)
- Synchronization between multiple systems
- Ordered patterning within a single system

Coherence is Different than Relaxation

It's important to explain why psycho-physiological coherence is a different state from relaxation. Coherence can include relaxation, but relaxation does not necessarily include heart coherence. In the coherence state, increased synchronization, resonance and entrainment between heart and brain and across multiple bodily systems occur—all of which reflect a level of global organization that is not present in the relaxation state alone. In terms of optimizing performance, it's important not to be too relaxed or overly stimulated. As we learn to maintain the coherence state, through sustaining sincere, heart-focused positive emotions (gratitude, care, kindness, love, etc.), our brain's electrical activity can come into increased synchronization with the heart. This activates our heart intelligence, which HeartMath founder Doc Childre defines as *"the flow of higher awareness, wisdom and intuition we experience when the mind and emotions are brought into synchronistic alignment with the heart."*

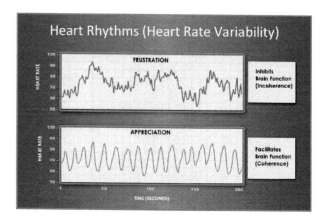

Relaxation has a different pattern in the heart rhythms and brain waves than coherence.

The Amygdala and the Thalamus

The heart rhythm pattern provides information about our emotional state to *the amygdala and the thalamus*. These brain centers are directly connected to the base of the frontal lobes and the executive centers of our brain, which are critical for decision making and the integration of reason and feeling. The thalamus synchronizes cortical activity, and is a pathway by which heart rhythms alter brainwave patterns and modify brain function. The signals from the heart travel to the amygdala by a different pathway.

The Amygdala

The amygdala is an emotional processing center and encodes emotional memories. The amygdala is also a pattern-matching system that scans for what's familiar. For example, when a stressful situation is perceived, the amygdala responds by scanning its memory banks until it finds the stored emotions from previous stressful experiences it assumes to be similar. Then it triggers the same emotional reactions we had last time – like anxiety, hurt, resignation or depression. The amygdala is able to "hijack" neural pathways and activate a familiar emotional response before our higher brain centers receive the information and before we have time to even "think" about how to respond. That's one reason we often react then say or do things we later regret. The amygdala communicates what is familiar to the perceptual centers in the brain. So if anger has become a familiar pattern to the amygdala, then perceiving someone looking at us strangely can trigger an anger reaction before we have time to consider whether anger is an appropriate response.

"Heart intelligence is the flow of awareness, wisdom and intuition we experience when the mind and emotions are brought into coherent alignment with the heart. It can be activated through self-initiated practice, and the more we pay attention when we sense the heart is speaking to us or guiding us, the greater our ability to access this intelligence and guidance more frequently. Heart intelligence underlies cellular organization and guides and evolves organisms toward increased order, awareness and coherence of their bodies' systems." **– Doc Childre**

Researchers know that survival programming deep in the brain causes the amygdala to put more weight on negative experiences than positive ones. The good news is that activating heart coherence and positive emotions, like equanimity, ease, compassion and gratitude, can encode new programming in the amygdala so that new more balanced and appropriate response patterns can be established. As you practice heart coherence, you set in place emotional patterns that will support you as you move forward in life and you release non-effective patterns. More of your real spirit comes in as mind and emotions are in coherent alignment with your heart. People can create a new familiar state and baseline, one that provides greater access to our full range of intelligence and unfolds "who we really are." The *HeartMath Brain Fitness Program* is designed to help us transform old survival programming and familiar reactions into heart intelligent perceptions and responses.

How does this work? The heart is primary player in establishing familiar patterns in the amygdala. The cells in the core of the amygdala are synchronized to the heart beat, due to the strong ascending neural pathway from the heart to the amygdala. This means if the rhythm of the heart is coherent, the amygdala will recognize that coherent rhythm. If your heart rhythm patterns are often disordered and incoherent, the amygdala learns to expect that incoherent rhythm; and thus we feel "at home" with incoherence, which compromises focus, emotional balance, learning and memory. Remember the amygdala (and the brain in general) is a pattern recognition and storage system and if we are stressed a lot, the amygdala recognizes stress as a familiar pattern. This is how we adapt to stress (a low grade feeling of anxiety or angst, irritability, etc.), which then becomes our new normal. A lot of people are afraid of letting go of old familiar moods. The familiar, even if it's miserable, is more comfortable. It's kind of like fish in a pond of dirty water. It's what is familiar and the fish have no perception that clean water even exists. This is how our subconscious emotional memories can affect our perceptions, emotional reactions, thought processes and behaviors.

The exciting news is that our emotional memory patterns can be re-ordered so that coherence becomes the more "familiar" and comfortable state. The heart can make the process of letting go of moods and habits that don't serve you quicker and easier. Practicing HeartMath techniques with heart rhythm coherence feedback helps establish coherence and increased emotional self-regulation as the familiar baseline, which improves our mental, emotional and physical health. We have more

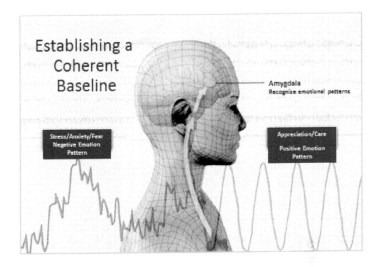

emotionally balanced responses and our brain can integrate reason and feeling to make more intelligent decisions. Heart coherence has been shown to facilitate working memory and attention, cortical processes, cognitive functions, creativity and performance. With regular practice, heart coherence becomes increasingly familiar to the brain. It takes on average 6–9 weeks of consistent practice of HeartMath tools and technology to establish new levels of emotional self-regulation and more coherent positive emotional baseline, which the brain then strives to maintain. The new skills can become automatic.

The Thalamus

The thalamus, a key brain center involved in optimal function, is also affected by the neural signals from the heart. One of the roles of the thalamus is to synchronize the neural activity of the entire brain, including the thinking part of our brain. This is important in understanding the relationship between emotional stability, mental functions and optimal performance. When we are feeling stress and our heart rhythm is incoherent, these rhythms impact the thalamus resulting in a desynchronization of cortical activity. These incoherent and chaotic rhythms interfere with the ability of the thalamus to synchronize cortical activity which has a global effect on the brain.

Desynchronization affects our frontal lobes the most. The frontal and pre-frontal cortex are where anything to do with planning or foresight takes place, as well as abstract thinking, problem-solving, creativity and discriminating appropriate behaviors (collectively called executive functions). For our frontal lobes to work well, they require very fine-tuned synchronized activity. When we intentionally shift into a coherent heart rhythm state, it facilitates these executive functions. When our heart rhythm is coherent, the thalamus is better able to synchronize cortical activity, and integrate the left and right hemispheres of the brain to see a bigger picture, providing the fine-tuned functioning we need.

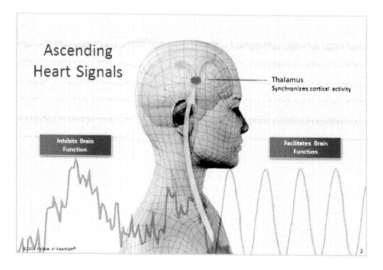

Self-Directedness and Leadership

Leadership starts with leading oneself or what noted psychiatrist Dr. Claude Robert Cloninger calls "self-directedness." Known for his pioneering research on the biological, psychological, social and spiritual foundation of mental health and mental illness he explains, "*Self-directedness involves being resourceful and confident that you can accomplish goals, being purposefully goal-directed, accepting yourself as you are with both strengths and weaknesses, being responsible rather than blaming, and eventually having cultivated good habits of self-regulation consistent with your goals and values. So it involves conscious development of emotional self-regulation or increasing choice, will, or internal locus of control free of past conditioning. Self-directedness allows people to keep the information coming into the brain from being blocked by alarm, anger, anxiety, so it can be maturely self-regulated. Self-directedness is correlated with the activation of the medial pre-frontal cortex in executive function tasks."*

The ability to quickly see both the whole and the key details of a situation is important for all of us. By seeing the "bigger picture," we are able to integrate disparate information coming to us from the environment, other people, and our own internal processes into a holistic framework of meaning that provides the basis for mental clarity and effective choices.

Coherence training is an optimal way to develop the capacity for greater self-directedness and to see the "bigger picture." It empowers us to replace negative emotions such as anger, anxiety and guilt with healthier emotions such as compassion, care or forgiveness, and shift our heart rhythm pattern on demand. As our brain and nervous system synchronize with our heart, the brain develops a familiar repository of healthy emotional responses from which it selects during times of stress. As heart coherence is practiced regularly, we actively create new neural patterns. Often within just 6–9 weeks, the brain and nervous system *rewire themselves to establish coherent heart rhythm patterns as a new baseline – the norm.* Much of our personal stress is created by anxious projections about what might happen (and often never does) or by frustration or anger about what has happened that we can't do anything about. Through coherence training, we can develop the heart power and intelligence to change that.

> "Since emotional processes can work faster than the mind, it takes a power stronger than the mind to bend perception, override emotional circuitry and provide us with intuitive feeling instead. It takes the power of the heart."
>
> **—Doc Childre, founder of HeartMath**

Focus and Attention

A recent article in the *New York Times* reported, "Brain scientists have discovered that swerving around cars while simultaneously picking out road signs in a video game can improve the short-term memory and long-term focus of older adults. Some people as old as 80, the researchers say, begin to show neurological patterns of people in their 20s. Cognitive scientists say the findings (published in the September 2013 issue of the scientific journal *Nature* called "Game Changer") are a significant development in understanding how to strengthen older brains. That is because the improvements in brain performance did not come just within the game but were shown outside the game in other cognitive tasks. Further supporting the findings, the researchers were able to measure and show changes in brain wave activity, suggesting that this research could help understand what neurological mechanisms should and could be tinkered with to improve memory and attention." Still, this research came with strong warnings from neuroscientists who find that the ability to maintain focus and attention is often made worse by technology because of constant stimulation and multi-tasking. Another study had found that people in their 20s experienced a 26 percent drop in performance when they were asked to multi-task by trying to drive and identify signs at the same time (rather than just identify the signs without driving). For people in their 60s to 80s, the performance drop was 64 percent.

HeartMath research has found that the ability to sustain attention is significantly enhanced when a self-generated positive emotional heart-coherent state is sustained. This has to do with how much interest or heart involvement we have in what we're doing. Since the heart's rhythmic pattern reflects our feelings and emotional experience, when we enjoy what we're doing the heart is instrumental in generating an outgoing wave of coherent energy. In other words, when we "put our heart" into what we are doing, we power up the mind and brain. Our heart is the energetically more powerful emotional component of focus and attention than mental (cognitive) attention alone.

Increasing Brain Power with Heart Power

Many organizations and health care systems have adopted HeartMath techniques and emWave technology to help their staff reduce stress, increase resilience and power-up performance. Health care professionals and surgeons tell us they take a few minutes to get into a heart coherent state before they see patients or do surgery, when they know they need their cognitive functions optimized. Heart coherence is like running higher octane gas through your system.

"If the brain were going to climb Mt. Everest, it needs the heart as the basecamp to climb from."
—**Doc Childre**

Meditation

Meditation has been shown to have positive effects on the brain and can help reverse memory loss as well as help improve psychological and spiritual well-being, which are both important for healthy brain aging. Meditation increases "presence" and "mindfulness" which is defined by Jon Kabat-Zinn author of Mindfulness-Based Stress Reduction (MBSR) books as "moment-to-moment, non-judgmental awareness, cultivated by paying attention in a specific way, that is, in the present moment, as non-reactively and non-judgmentally as possible." According to our friend, Dr. Daniel Siegel, author of the book *Mindsight,* meditation can help our brains achieve a state of "integration" that lends itself to social and emotional well-being.

Using the emWave or Inner Balance technology takes the economy of meditation to a new level. The instant feedback and realignment it gives us results in increased coherence (integration) and effectiveness in shorter periods of time. Most of us really need that because of the fast pace of the world with all the things we have to do and limited time to meditate. The emWave or Inner Balance technology will clinically give you more economy in the meditation process. You get a lot more for doing less, which we all need these days.

"Using the emWave literally gives you 'more bang for the buck' in a shorter period of time -- and you're still the one doing it. It's not the machine doing it, but what a meditation buddy it is." —**Doc Childre**

Part III – Sharpen your Brain with Your Heart

There are many brain fitness programs, games, exercises, puzzles, assessments and devices. *The SharpBrains Guide to Brain Fitness* did a good job investigating and reviewing many of these. The HeartMath Brain Fitness Program can be added to any of them to help power-up and increase their effectiveness. Heart-brain synchronization will add balance and coherence to any program and is often the missing link to improving or sustaining outcomes. You can also use the HeartMath Brain Fitness Program by itself, and you will likely achieve results similar to those described in Part IV.

HeartMath Brain Fitness Five Step Program

1. Learn and practice the Neutral and Quick Coherence® techniques
2. Learn to Operate your emWave or Inner Balance Trainer
3. Practice the Quick Coherence technique with your emWave or Inner Balance Trainer
4. Sustain Coherence with the Heart Lock-In® Technique
5. Use the Freeze Frame® technique to Improve Decision-Making and Creativity

Step 1—Learn and Practice the Neutral and Quick Coherence techniques

Using the Neutral technique will help you bring your mind, emotions and nervous system to a state of "neutral." This technique is especially helpful when you want to slow or stop an energy draining reaction. Many people use the Neutral technique 10–20 times a day and find it saves a lot of energy—and saves them from saying or doing something from a reactive place that they may later regret. The technique is simple and can be done anytime, anywhere.

Neutral Technique

Heart-Focused Breathing. Focus your attention in the area of the heart. Imagine your breath is flowing in and out of your heart or chest area, breathing a little slower and deeper than usual. *Suggestion. Inhale 5 seconds, exhale 5 seconds (or whatever rhythm is comfortable).*

Practice the Neutral technique when you're reacting or stuck in a negative view of a situation. As you do Heart-Focused Breathing, tell yourself, "Take out the drama," and ask yourself, "Do I really want to drain energy over this?," and "What if there is more to the picture than you can know at this time?" Asking yourself these questions from a sincere heart can help you shift into neutral more quickly and be open to new information.

Quick Coherence Technique

Step 1. Focus your attention in the area of the heart. Imagine your breath is flowing in and out of your heart or chest area, breathing a little slower and deeper than usual. *Suggestion. Inhale 5 seconds, exhale 5 seconds (or whatever rhythm is comfortable)*

Step 2. Make a sincere attempt to experience a regenerative feeling such as appreciation or care for someone or something in your life.
Suggestion. Try to re-experience the feeling you have for someone you love, a pet, a special place, an accomplishment, etc., or focus on a feeling of calm or ease.

Quick Coherence Quick Steps.

Step 1. Heart-Focused Breathing
Step 2. Activate a positive or renewing feeling

Practice the Quick Coherence technique to release stress or anxiety and learn to shift into a positive emotional state or more balanced attitude by choice. Observe any changes in perception that follow. You can take a 30-second coherence break anytime with your eyes open—between activities, at your desk, walking down the hall, on a break or anywhere. Simply shift focus to your heart (look at picture of a loved one, remember a favorite pet or recall a time in nature) and feel appreciation or gratitude. It's important that the appreciation be heartfelt (not just from the mind) to activate heart coherence and the hormones that help bring balance and harmony to your mental and emotional processes. Breathe a genuine feeling or attitude of appreciation through the area of your heart for a minute (without mentally multi-tasking as you do this). Taking coherence breaks builds resilience and helps you listen to your heart's intuitive guidance on what else you need to do to prevent or release stress build-up and find more ease and flow in your mind and emotions throughout the day.

Step 2—Learn to Operate your emWave or Inner Balance technology

The SharpBrains Guide to Brain Fitness investigated the emWave Desktop (also called emWave Pro) technology. The emWave Desktop uses either an ear sensor or finger sensor connected to a USB module running on emWave software. It monitors and displays your heart rhythm pattern and your coherence level on a computer screen. This multi-user technology automatically records and stores each user's session so they can track their progress over time. The emWave Desktop includes: 1) An application called the Coherence Coach®, which guides you in the Quick Coherence technique and uses a breathing pacer to help you synchronize your breathing, emotions and heart rhythms. 2) Several beautiful emotion visualizers and three colorful interactive games that respond to your coherence level and add layers of fun and novelty to the overall training experience.

The emWave2 is a handheld single user portable device that has many of the same functions as the emWave Desktop. It displays your heart rhythm pattern and coherence level in colored lights and comes with a software CD that includes the Coherence Coach, one emotion visualizer and one game. The emWave2 stores your data so you can sync it with the software and view your sessions and your progress on your computer.

The Inner Balance is emWave technology in an iOS app that you use with your iPhone, iPad or iPod Touch. You plug in the Inner Balance sensor to the charger port of your iOS device.

In order to use *HeartMath Brain Fitness Program,* you need to become familiar with how to operate your emWave or your Inner Balance technology.

- Remove the sensor and contents from the box and read the instructions. We recommend you take the short e-training program for the product you have www.emwavetraining.com and/or attend the 1-hour telephone orientation class offered each week.
- Attach the pulse sensor to the fleshy part of your ear lobe and move it around until you get a good pulse signal on your device. Explore the different functions on your emWave or Inner Balance Trainer and get comfortable using it.

Step 3—Practice the Quick Coherence technique while using your emWave or Inner Balance Trainer.

Once you have learned the Quick Coherence technique, you are ready to use it along with your device. While connected to the emWave or Inner Balance device, slowly practice the steps of the Quick Coherence technique. Imagine the breath going in through the area of the heart and out through the area of the heart. Synchronize your breathing with the breath pacer on your device. Watch the changes in your heart rhythm. If the pacer is going too fast or too slow you can change the speed in your settings to something more comfortable. Generally practicing Heart-Focused Breathing to a count of 5 or 6 on the in breath and a count of 5 or 6 on the out breath will start to increase your coherence.

Your goal in using the Quick Coherence technique with the technology is to get the red light on your emWave (red dot on your Inner Balance) to turn from red (low coherence) which is normal, to blue (medium coherence) which is much improved, to green (high coherence) which is the optimal high performance state. Genuine heartfelt appreciation or gratitude is often the easiest positive emotion to find and quickly shifts the heart rhythm into coherence. Sustain blue or green as long as you can. Make it a gentle process and continue to feel appreciation. If you do the technique with your eyes closed, which can be helpful when you are first learning, you'll be able to tell when you have shifted into medium or high coherence through listening to the change in audio tones if you have the sound turned on.

If you are easily achieving high coherence scores – at least 80% in the green then increase the challenge level. If you have a score of 80% or more in the red, spend more focused time with the Coherence Coach®. Low scores are normal at the beginning, but with practice, they will improve. As scores improve, you can go up to the next challenge level; there are four levels. If you have an em-Wave Desktop, once you become proficient at a basic level, you can try some of the fun emotion visualizers and the coherence games. A score of 50% or more in blue (medium coherence) is required to play the software games. Start with the three-minute Garden Game. Then move on to the five-minute Rainbow Game. If progress has been made, try the 10-minute Balloon Game. You can use the Emotion Visualizer® to add variety to your training sessions.

Using your emWave or Inner Balance several times each day will help you maintain or regain balance, calm and composure, while reducing fatigue. Many mental health professionals promote "downtime" or taking mental breaks during "in-between moments" during the day— between meetings, at lunch, before a next project, etc. This is because key brain processes seem to require short periods of rest, meditation or thought quieting "downtime" practices to refresh the ability to remain attentive, stay motivated or engaged and achieve higher levels of performance. HeartMath research has found that the quality and effectiveness of "downtime" can be achieved in less time and the outcomes enhanced with heart coherence practice. Getting in high coherence (in the green) even for a few minutes can quickly align your heart and brain to bring you important perception shifts, so you can see a larger picture or find new solutions to time pressures or stressful issues that you couldn't see before.

Prep and Reset

There are times during the day that you'll especially want to use Quick Coherence with your emWave or Inner Balance heart coherence technology and "get in the green" to prep for a potentially stressful upcoming event or to reset your heart and brain after a stressful experience. It's easy when stressed to think you're back in balance when you're not. That's why it's important to get the real-time coherence feedback so that you know when you really have made the shift. The technology keeps you honest and on track and accelerates your ability to shift into coherence and establish a new neural habit.

* Times to Prep (prepare) for potentially stressful events
    * First thing in the morning before you start your workday
    * Before a commute where you are likely to face traffic jams
    * Before going to speak with someone you know could be difficult or before speaking to a group of people when your mind could jam
    * Before a meeting that could be challenging.
    * Before responding to an email that you reacted to.
    * Before any situation that is likely to trigger your emotions

* Times to Reset (recover) from stressful episodes
    * After a difficult conversation when you are stressing over what was said or what you should have said
    * After feeling overloaded by work or time pressure

- After feeling anxious about something that didn't go the way you wanted
- After anything that triggered you emotionally

The Carryover Effect

Using emWave or Inner Balance to prep or reset has a profound *carryover* effect. As you practice sitting in coherence, it adds energy to your system and opens a connection to your heart's intuitive guidance that carries over into your next perceptions and choices.

The accumulation of coherence in your mental and emotional system carries over into your activities and interactions, even when you're not walking around in high coherence (in the green). It gives you more objectivity to make better decisions. You'll find it's easier to let go of irritations and regain inner balance. It's easier to be patient, to listen more deeply, to move with ease and find a flow in your communications.

The more often you use the Quick Coherence technique and "get in the green" with the technology, the quicker you will be able to change your stress set point. And as you learn to clear stress as you go, you reduce the amount of cortisol (stress hormone) you are adding to your system, which can help you think more clearly and improve your memory.

Sometimes it's harder to quiet the mind. You may have what are called "recurring thought loops" about a person or situation. Your mind rehashes a situation and your emotions react to what you are thinking with worry, anger or other stressful feeling. These stressful thoughts and feelings generate incoherence in your heart's rhythms and make it much harder to function or have optimal performance. The second HeartMath technique you will learn in Step 4, called the Heart Lock-In technique helps you sustain coherence for longer periods and helps release stubborn recurring mental and emotional loops.

Step 4—Practice Sustaining Coherence with the Heart Lock-In®Technique

You can practice the Heart Lock-in technique with your emWave or Inner Balance technology instead of the Quick Coherence technique in the morning to help sustain the carryover effect into your workday or as part of a meditation routine to improve focus and connection with your deeper self. You can also use the Heart Lock-In technique with your technology before bed to assist in more restful sleep. *Turn on the audio and let the tones guide you into coherence and help you sustain coherence.

Heart Lock-In Technique

Step 1. Focus your attention in the area of the heart. Imagine your breath is flowing in and out of your heart or chest area, breathing a little slower and deeper than usual.

Step 2. Activate and sustain a regenerative feeling such as appreciation, care or compassion.

Step 3. Radiate that renewing feeling to yourself and others.

Heart Lock-In Quick Steps

Step 1. Heart-Focused Breathing

Step 2. Activate a regenerative Feeling

Step 3. Radiate that Feeling

Just radiate positive feelings from the heart. Gently feel as if these positive emotions are going out to others, to the world, or to you. If stressful thoughts or preoccupations try to take over, bring your focus and your breathing gently back to the area around the heart. Try to feel a caring softness in your heart area and reconnect with feelings of care, appreciation or gratitude for someone or something in your life.

Practice the Heart Lock in technique with your emWave or Inner Balance for 10 to 15 minutes at Challenge Level 1. (If you are using emWave

*For instructions on how to use your emWave or Inner Balance device to improve sleep, see the emWave and Inner Balance Solution for Better Sleep.

> **Cynthia Pearsall, Chief Nursing Officer, at Fairfield Medical Center and a certified HeartMath trainer describes how she uses Heart Lock-In.**
>
> "When you feel stressed", she explains "you can literally flip the switch anytime, anyplace, into the 'stress free zone' by changing the instant message the heart sends to the brain by way of the nervous system." I start every day with a HeartMath technique called "Heart Lock-In" to strengthen my ability to sustain a coherent state, to achieve balance and synchronization between my heart and mind, and to become more resilient to the stresses I am sure to face throughout the day. I even begin all of my meetings this way, with a 90-second Heart Lock-in; and if we are having a difficult time reaching a decision as a team, I will ask each of us to take a couple minutes to practice some easy coherence steps to change the quality of the moment. Once the meeting resumes, we can reliably reach a decision. HeartMath is bringing this family of caregivers, indeed this local community, closer together."

Desktop or emWave Pro, do a 10–15 min session at your computer before going to bed.) Turn on the audio tone to guide you into coherence (unless it will bother someone else) so you can close your eyes. If you find it very easy to stay in high coherence, you can move to Challenge Level 2 which will help you further increase coherence in your heart rhythm pattern.

Spending a little time in a Heart Lock-In feeling positive emotions is extremely beneficial for mental, emotional and physical health and healing. Genuinely felt positive emotions that help increase heart-brain synchronization a include love, care, appreciation, compassion, kindness, tolerance, patience, ease, peace and more. You can spend time in a Heart Lock-in exploring these feelings and seeing how they affect your coherence levels.

Studies have found many benefits from learning positive emotional self-regulation. Positive psychology researcher Barbara Fredrickson says, "Positive emotions can have effects beyond making people 'feel good'

Benefits of Positive Emotions

> Increased longevity (Danner et al., 2001)

> Increased resilience to adversity (Frederickson et al., 2003)

> Increased cognitive flexibility (Ashby et al., 1999)

> Improved memory (Isen et al., 1978)

> Increased immune function (Rein et al., 1995, McCraty et al., 1996)

> Improved problem solving (Carnevale & Isen, 1986)

> Increased intuition and creativity (Bolte et al., 2003; Isen et al., 1987)

> Increased happiness (Frederickson & Joiner, 2002)

> Improved job performance and achievement
(Wright & Staw, 1994; Staw et al., 1994)

or improving their subjective experiences of life. They also have the potential to broaden people's habitual modes of thinking and build their physical, intellectual and social resources. In addition, these resources last longer than the transient positive emotional states that led to their acquisition and can be drawn upon in future moments, when people are in different emotional states, to help them overcome current stresses faster and make them more resilient to future adversities."

Step 5: Use the Freeze Frame technique to Improve Decision-Making and Creativity

We are all decision-makers, making a staggering number of both big and small decisions each day. In today's fast pace of life, we can be faced with making important decisions quickly and often without having all the information we would like or need. By slowing down your inner mental and emotional responses with the Freeze Frame technique, you create a time-out that allows you to think more clearly from a more balanced, intuitive and coherent perspective.

More often however, we do not have to make "big" decisions in the heat of the moment. Likely, though, there is a constant stream of choices we have to make throughout the day that can have significant short- and long-term consequences. Some of these may be more important than others and some more emotionally charged than others. Bigger decisions take focus, consideration of information and opinions, and some have to be made with a good bit of intuition. Some of the decisions whether personal or professional can create a low-grade anxiety.

Our attitudes and feelings about people, situations and issues are always involved in our decisions, often under the radar. It's common to have selective memory, remembering only emotionally charged issues around a person or event, so it's imperative to clear the screen so we can make more objective and appropriate decisions and bring in our heart intelligence to provide a synthesis of information stored in memory, new information we may have not thought of, and our intuitive sense.

By practicing the simple Freeze Frame technique, we can quickly get our physiology (brain and nervous system) in sync to help clear the screen and access our heart intelligence before making decisions, big or small.

The Freeze Frame technique helps to balance and integrate mind, heart, emotions and intuition. This technique allows you to use more of your smart-thinking brain, which gets jammed up and out of sync during angry, anxious, worried or confused states. It's important to remember the role the heart's rhythms play in this process. When the heart's rhythms are chaotic or incoherent (reflecting an out-of-sync nervous system), they inhibit or limit your ability to think clearly, reason, remember and stay focused. But when you shift your heart rhythm into a smooth and flowing pattern, it enhances your brain's abilities. It aligns your heart, mind and emotions and connects you with your heart's intuitive guidance.

You can use the Freeze Frame technique and worksheet to quickly move from recognizing a problem or stressful issue to finding a solution that can be put into action. You can also use the Freeze Frame technique for accessing creative ideas or intuitive insights on projects you are planning or engaged in. The more you increase your coherence baseline, the more access you will have to your creative capacities.

The Steps of FREEZE FRAME®

Step 1. *Acknowledge* the problem or issue and any attitudes or feelings about it.

It's important to be honest with yourself about what you are feeling, whether it is frustration, annoyance, anxiety, impatience, fear, anger or something else. You can write down how you have been mentally and emotionally feeling about the issue to gain more honest clarity.

Step 2. Focus your attention in the area of the heart. Imagine your breath is flowing in and out of your heart or chest area, breathing a little slower and deeper than usual. *Suggestion. Inhale 5 second, exhale 5 seconds (or whatever rhythm is comfortable)*

This step lets you take a time-out, which allows you to disengage from any stressful feelings and brings your system into a state of Neutral. This allows you to freeze the frame — isolate the moment.

Remember, combining the simple act of focusing on the heart area with a deeper level of breathing helps draw energy away from incoherent, confused or distressed thoughts and feelings and into a state of Neutral.

Step 3. Make a sincere attempt to experience a regenerative feeling such as appreciation or care for someone or something in your life.

You want to try to experience a regerative feeling. Remember a posi-tive moment. Re-experience the feeling of it. It is the sincere feeling that comes from the experience that counts and creates more coherence in your body's systems. Together, Steps 2 and 3 create more coherence, which facilitates the higher mental functions and intuitive insights.

Step 4. From this more objective place, ask yourself what would be a more efficient or effective attitude, action or solution.

When you ask yourself, the coherence created in steps 2 and 3 enable higher mental functions and intuitive insights that typically are compromised during stressful or challenging situations. You have greater ability to think clearly and objectively, and the issue, interaction or decision now can be viewed from a broader, more emotionally balanced and intelligent perspective.

Step 5. Quietly observe any subtle changes in perceptions, attitudes or feelings. Commit to sustaining beneficial attitude shifts and acting on new insights.

Freeze Frame Quick Steps.
- **Step 1.** Acknowledge
- **Step 2.** Heart-Focused Breathing
- **Step 3.** Activate a positive or renewing feeling
- **Step 4.** Ask
- **Step 5.** Observe and Act

It's helpful to write down whatever you observe to help you remember it. This will also help you develop the important skill of listening to your deeper self — your intuition, or heart feelings. A major source of depletion results from either not connecting with or ignoring our intuitive intelligence. Try to remain focused in the heart area. (This will help you maintain coherence during the process and keep you from jumping back into thought loops that can block your intuitions.) You may observe new insights, different attitudes or feelings that may help you deal with the problem or issue or have more creative ideas— a coherent response. Many people find that their emWave or Inner Balance turns green (high coherence) when they have a new attitude or insight.

It's okay if no insights come up, remember shifting how you feel about it reduces stress, too. Be patient with yourself as you learn these steps. Repeat the process later or the next day. It will begin to feel more natural with practice. For some issues, it is harder to find clarity. This has a lot to do with the complexity of the issue, past history and the intensity of any emotions that may or not be related to the issue or situation.

Action Plan

Practice of the Freeze Frame technique with the emWave or Inner Balance app will help establish new neural activity patterns in the brain and nervous system, where more coherent and clear perceptions and decisions become easier, in both large and small choices you make, saving you time and energy and bringing more reward.

An executive in a Fortune 100 high tech company describes using the Freeze Frame technique: *"I think of it as a business power-tool. After using the Freeze Frame® technique in my work for a couple of years, I find it indispensable for creative planning, problem-solving, making clear decisions and maintaining a high level of stamina during long days. I'm able to gain access to more clear, creative and intelligent solutions. My work throws me into lots of situations that I have to plan for but can't control. This tool has helped me generate creative solutions in unexpected situations that required clear 'thinking on my feet.' A side effect of using Freeze Frame at work is it's nice to have some energy and creativity to take home with me at the end of a long day!"*

You can use Freeze Frame worksheets to help you learn the skill.

Freeze Frame Worksheet

The Steps of FREEZE FRAME®

Step 1. Acknowledge the problem or issue and any attitudes or feelings about it.

Step 2. Focus your attention in the area of the heart. Imagine your breath is flowing in and out of your heart or chest area, breathing a little slower and deeper than usual. Suggestion. Inhale 5 second, exhale 5 seconds (or whatever rhythm is comfortable)

Step 3. Make a sincere attempt to experience a regenerative feeling such as appreciation or care for someone or something in your life.

Step 4. From this more objective place, ask yourself what would be a more efficient or effective attitude, action or solution.

Step 5. Quietly observe any subtle changes in perceptions, attitudes or feelings. Commit to sustaining beneficial attitude shifts and acting on new insights.

Problem or Issue:

Attitudes and feelings about the issue:

Practice the Freeze Frame Steps

What did you observe?

Before: _____ After: _____

Often, solutions are inspired through communicating or getting input from others.

Worksheet Instructions:

It's a good idea when you are first learning the technique to practice on a smaller issue or decision. Go step by step. Don't be surprised if the insight you get seems simple or too easy or you have a change in how you feel about the situation. A coherent response comes when you quiet the mind chatter and take out the emotional reactivity.

Step 1 is to first acknowledge an issue or problem that is causing some stress in your life or that you need more clarity about before making a decision.

Write down the stressor or issue on the worksheet. Next take a couple of minutes and reflect on the thoughts and feelings you have been having around the situation or issue. Be honest with yourself about your thoughts and feelings, whether they include confusion, overwhelm, frustration, annoyance, anxiety, impatience, fear or something else. Write them down in the space provided on the worksheet. Notice what you experience revisiting this issue or problem.

Now go through the remaining steps of Freeze Frame.

Step 2 is Heart-Focused Breathing.

Step 3, attempt to experience a regerative feeling. You want to try and feel a positive emotion. Relive a positive moment, one in which you felt good, and re-experience it. It's the sincere feeling that comes from the experience that counts and creates coherence. For example, it might be the good feeling that comes from hanging out with friends, having accomplished a goal or watching a sunset. Don't just visualize it. Try to feel it.

Step 4, ask yourself what a more efficient attitude or approach to the issue or situation may be.

Step 5, it is important to develop the skill of listening to your intuition or heart. A major source of depletion results from ignoring your own intuitive intelligence. Quietly observe any subtle thoughts, feelings or perceptions that you have about the decision, situation or issue. Write down any changes in perception or any new insights in the space provided on the worksheet. If you did not gain any clarity, but felt differently, e.g. calmer, that is a change. You may want to revisit the issue and do another Freeze Frame exercise. You can also start with whatever answer you wrote down as the issue, and then go through the steps again to deepen or gain more understanding. With practice, Freeze Framing will become a very natural process that you can do on the spot to access the appropriate response in many situations.

Summary of the Five Step Program

1. Learn and practice the Neutral and Quick Coherence techniques.

- Learn to use Heart-Focused Breathing to shift into Neutral to stop energy draining reactions and to use Quick Coherence to shift into a positive coherent state. You'll use these two in-the-moment tools more often if you also practice with your eyes open.

2. Learn to Operate your emWave or Inner Balance Trainer

3. Practice the Quick Coherence technique with your emWave or Inner Balance Trainer.

- Prep" before a potentially stressful situation and "Reset" quickly after a stressful experience.

- Get in medium coherence (blue) then high coherence (green) and stay in high coherence for a few minutes to increase the carryover effect.

- Use your device 3–4 times/day even if you think you don't need to. Sometimes you're not in coherence when you think you are and the feedback shows you that, and you go deeper.

- Sitting in high coherence on the emWave or playing a coherence game on the emWave Desktop or emWave2 several times per day can create new neural patterns in 6–9 weeks.

4. Practice Sustaining Coherence with the Heart Lock-In Technique.

- Use the Heart Lock-in technique with your emWave or Inner Balance and "get in the green" for 10–15 minutes to sustain coherence for longer periods and increase your coherence baseline.

5. Use the Freeze Frame technique to Improve decision-making and creativity.

- Use the Freeze Frame technique for problem-solving, to gain more intuitive insight on an issue or a project, and for intuitive decision-making.

This Program works best if you practice daily. There will be modulations where some days it's easier to get into heart rhythm coherence than others. This can be due to extra stress accumulation, changing biorhythms or hormones, or even solar flares and geomagnetic activity. That's when you want to reduce the challenge level and know that you are still receiving the benefits. You are still making progress as it's the practice that counts. Be patient and compassionate with yourself. Remember it usually takes six to nine weeks of consistent practice to reset a neural pattern.

Part IV – HeartMath Brain Fitness Outcomes

Since the mid 1990's HeartMath training programs in schools, organizations, health care systems and the military have repeatedly been shown to improve cognitive function and empower behavior change. Improvements have been observed in maintaining focus and concentration, problem solving, emotional self-regulation and abstract thinking. Improvements in cognitive functions were also achieved in tasks requiring discrimination and fast reactions, coordination, accuracy and performance in various sports. Research from the Institute of HeartMath has demonstrated that heart coherence training enabled reduced test anxiety and higher test scores in school and college settings, better ability to learn, and increased ability to focus and process information. For example, one college mathematics readiness program that found that incorporating the emWave and HeartMath self-regulation techniques in college classes increased math scores by 73% in one semester, when use of the techniques was integrated into the classroom learning on a regular basis.

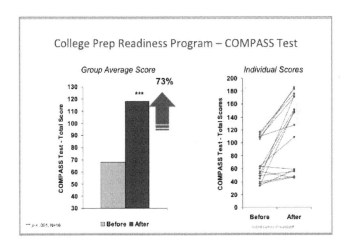

Reaction Times

An important measure of brain fitness is "reaction time." Thirty participants were randomly divided into matched control and experimental groups based on age and gender in this study. Cognitive performance was assessed by determining their reaction times in an auditory discrimination task before and after practicing the Heart Lock-In technique to increase their heart rhythm coherence. After the practice of the Heart Lock-In, the participants were instructed to push a button as quickly as possible whenever they heard the "odd" tones, which were randomly interspaced in between the standard tone. (The control group engaged in a relaxation period instead of practicing the Heart Lock-In technique before and after the auditory discrimination task.) Heart rhythm coherence, derived from the ECG, was calculated for all participants during each phase of the testing sequence. As shown in the graph below, there was a significant improvement in reaction times in the Heart Lock-In group and no change in the control group.

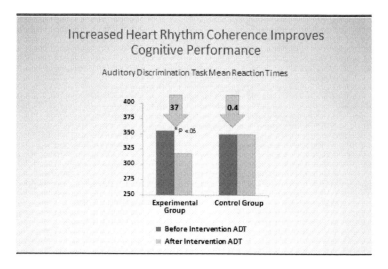

Reducing Mistakes

A multi-billion-dollar US grocery chain with 200+ in-store pharmacies provided a HeartMath stress and performance intervention with the portable emWave2 technology for heart-brain synchronization to a pilot group of their pharmacists. Measures of prescription error rate were tracked along with a survey to capture stress levels, and job as well as home life satisfaction. The objective was to reduce stress, manage incident rate, and promote happier, healthier and more satisfied employees. The initial pilot included 70 pharmacists. Results were excellent in all areas, including a 40% reduction in prescription errors. A second program with 152 pharmacists resulted in significantly improved wellness data and a 40–71% reduction in prescription errors.

Behavior Change

Behavioral specialists use the HeartMath self-regulation techniques and heart coherence feedback technologies to help adults and children address behavioral challenges such as anger management, interpersonal conflict and communication. Many special education classrooms employ the emWave Desktop in their computer labs to help students learn the techniques to gain greater impulse control, academic focus and confidence, and be more actively engage in the learning process.

Organizations often provide HeartMath training programs and technology to employees to manage stress and sustain resilience and focus in the face of challenging job demands and long hours. Pre- and Post-assessments (Personal and Organizational Quality Assessment - POQA) of nearly 10,000 employees found that, in just 6 to 9 weeks, HeartMath training consistently improved mental health factors and reduced personal stress, including a 50% drop in fatigue, 46% drop in anxiety, 60% drop in depression and 30% improvement in sleep along with significant improvements in strategic understanding, goal clarity and work attitude. Furthermore, post-assessments 6 months and 12 months after HeartMath trainings showed sustained mental health improvements, The POQA's Organizational Quality scales examine key areas that influence employee job involvement, performance and important factors related to employee behavior and ability to perform well. These include: freedom of expression, confidence in the organization, job challenge, value of contribution, communication effectiveness, manager support, morale, work intensity, productivity, time pressure and intention to quit. These areas also showed significant improvements, including a 41% reduction in intent to leave the job, 24% improvement in the ability to focus, 25% improvement in listening ability and 17% improvement in home/work conflict. All of this adds up to increased performance and satisfaction, improved health and cost savings to the organization.

Training in HeartMath helped The California Public Employees' Retirement System (CalPERS) employees effectively transform an environment of emotional turmoil that had developed in response to the implementation of major organizational change. Compared to an untrained comparison group, employees who learned HeartMath tools experienced significant reductions in anger, anxiety, distress, depression, sadness, fatigue and physical stress symptoms. Trained employees also demonstrated significant increases in productivity, goal clarity, peacefulness and vitality relative to the comparison group.

Employees of the Canadian Imperial Bank of Commerce trained in the Freeze Frame technique showed an extremely high level of retention and consistent application of the technique both in business and personal life one year after the training. Employees placed high value on the Freeze Frame technique, with most feeling it significantly affected their behavior and improved their overall well-being.

Police officers trained in the HeartMath tools experienced decreased stress, negative emotions and fatigue, increased calmness and clarity under the acute stress of simulated police calls, and more rapid recalibration following these high-stress scenarios, as compared to a control group. Trained officers also demonstrated improvements in work performance, communication and cooperation at work, and relationships with family after learning and practicing the tools.

ADD/ADHD

Attention Deficit Disorder (ADD) and Attention Deficit Hyperactivity disorder (ADHD) are a growing concern in children and adults. Mental health professionals use HeartMath techniques and techology to help adults and children deal with symptoms of ADD/ADHD, as well as anger management, anxiety, depression, autism, traumatic brain injury and other mental challenges.

ADHD is one of the most common childhood developmental problems and is characterized by inattention, hyperactivity and impulsiveness. It is now known that these symptoms continue into adulthood for about 60% of children with ADHD. However, few adults are identified or treated for ADHD. ADHD can make it hard for adults to pay attention, control their emotions, and finish tasks. In these days of information overload, time pressure and multi-tasking, many more adults are developing symptoms of ADD/ ADHD. People with ADD/ADHD may have difficulty following directions, remembering information, concentrating, organizing tasks, or completing work within time limits. If these difficulties are not managed appropriately, they can cause behavioral, emotional, social, career and academic problems.

The following behaviors and problems may stem directly from ADHD or may be the result of related adjustment difficulties.

- Anxiety
- Chronic boredom
- Chronic lateness and forgetfulness
- Depression
- Difficulty concentrating when reading
- Difficulty controlling anger
- Employment problems
- Substance abuse or addiction

- Impulsiveness
- Low frustration tolerance
- Low self-esteem
- Mood swings
- Poor organization skills
- Procrastination
- Relationship problems

Children and adults diagnosed with ADHD are often given stimulant drugs or other medications to control symptoms but there are other effective treatments. Dr. Daniel Amen, author *Change Your Brain, Change your Life* and Dr. Edward Hallowell author of *Driven to Distraction: Recognizing and*

Coping with Attention Deficit Disorder (and other books on brain health), are pioneers in natural treatments including diet, nutritional supplements, exercise, brain games and biofeedback and are friends of HeartMath. Heart rhythm coherence feedback has been utilized in ADHD studies.

In one study, a randomized controlled clinical trial in England evaluated the impact of the HeartMath emotional self-regulation skills and coherence feedback training on a population of 38 children with ADHD in academic year groups 6, 7, and 8. Fourteen children were in the experimental group and twenty four children in the placebo-controlled group for the first six weeks and then were given the same HeartMath intervention the Experimental group received during the next six weeks. Legos were chosen as an active placebo for the control group, as Legos are used as a therapeutic method for children with ADHD. The experimental group learned and practiced three HeartMath coherence techniques for six weeks: Neutral, Quick Coherence and Heart Lock-In techniques. Learning HeartMath techniques was supported with heart rhythm coherence monitoring and feedback with the emWave Desktop.

A computerized cognitive function assessment was used to assess a wide range of cognitive functions. Other outcome measures assessed teacher and student reported changes in behavior. The participants using HeartMath skills demonstrated significant improvements in number of cognitive functions, such as delayed word recall (long-term memory), immediate word recall (short-term memory), word recognition, and vigilance (focus and concentration). Significant improvements in behavior were also found. The data showed that these improvements were not gained at the expense of speed. The results were significantly beyond what was expected. The results suggest that the HeartMath intervention offers a physiologically based program to improve cognitive functioning in children with ADHD and improve behaviors that are appropriate to implement in a school environment. (Coherence Training in Children With ADHD: Cognitive Functions and Behavioral Changes, conducted by Anthony Lloyd, Ph.D., David.Brett,.BSc, Keith Wesnes, Ph.D.

Study Design

- 38 Students
- 6th and 7th Grade
- 3 Academic Centres
- Placebo controlled positive research paradigm
- Primary Hypothesis:
  - "Coherence training improves cognitive function, post training, to a significance $p > 0.05$ in the intervention group"

Summary of Results

- Immediate word recall improved 24%
- Delayed word recall improved 45%
- Word Recognition improved 28%
- Vigilance improved 9.5%

Observational Results

- Improved sleeping patterns
- Improved relationships with siblings
- Reduction in oppositional behaviour – Home
- Reported improvements in self confidence
- Reduction in oppositional behaviour – school

ADHD and Arrhythmia

Dr. Shari St. Martin taught a program sponsored by the University of Guadalajara in Mexico, similar to a program she taught in Marin County California schools with high intelligence children who had ADD/ADHD. She also opened a clinic in Guadalajara to help treat children with ADD/ADHD. Dr. St. Martin used the first version of emWave Desktop (formerly called the Freeze-Framer®) with children ranging from 6 to 18 years in age. By using heart rhythm coherence feedback, to support learning of the self-regulation skills, she made a surprising discovery: that a majority of the children were suffering from cardiac arrhythmias (verified by a local cardiologist). This finding pointed to a clear psycho-physiological factor that could contribute to the manifestation of the symptoms of ADD/ADHD.

Dr. St. Martin introduced the children to the emWave Desktop games that operate on the user's coherence level: Balloon Game, Rainbow Game and Meadow Game. She wrote, *"The responses were sometimes challenging because the children would have to work with their feelings and emotions, something they were not accustomed to; however, they quickly grew to feel that they had a safe place in which to practice the heart coherence techniques without judgment. The children soon felt free to move the balloon or the rainbow or to color the meadow by just feeling or tapping into their emotions. It was especially empowering when they were able to complete one of the games successfully and then view their heart rhythm coherence scores, which showed a stable and highly coherent heart rhythm. Being able to create the images on the screen through their own emotional management skills and improving their heart rhythm coherence scores each time gave the children a sense of high self-esteem and generated feelings of self-empowerment."*

At the time of writing her report, Dr. St. Martin had used emWave Desktop with 396 children with ADD/ADHD. She evaluated the improvements in the children's ability to self-regulate their emotions by using the HeartMath tools with feedback and found that the HeartMath tools combined with the technology also helped correct the cardiac arrhythmia. The improvements gained were so profound that they eliminated the need for ADHD-related medication in the vast majority of the children she worked with. It was also discovered that some children were taking too much stimulant medication and when taken off the meds (approved by their physicians) due to behavioral improvements from using HeartMath technology, their arrhythmia was reduced. The mother of one child had shared her disappointment and frustration with her son's stealing, lying, and passive-aggressive behavior as well as his diagnosis of ADHD. After the ninth session of working with this child with the HeartMath techniques and emWave games, the boy's mother reported that there was no more lying or stealing and that her son had changed drastically. He was more sociable and more compassionate toward his parents and others. His academic scores had also significantly improved and he felt much more relaxed and secure about himself.

The Falcone Institute specializes in helping youth address academic difficulties, neurological disabilities, depression and family conflict. It has used the emWave Desktop technology for years to help clients manage stress.

"With children who are diagnosed with ADHD, the staff at the Falcone Institute first makes sure there has not been a misdiagnosis. Occasionally with ADHD diagnoses, there has been unrecognized trauma or other secondary causes which manifest ADHD-like symptoms in a child. Diagnostic assessments from a pediatrician or developmental psychologist are reviewed to make sure the profile is accurate. In addition, several exercises are carried out with the child to see if the typical symptoms of impulsivity, inattentiveness and hyperactivity show up.

"After the diagnosis is confirmed, the child is then exposed to a series of structured activities to help with greater self-control. This includes using the

---

*If you are working with children with ADHD, see the HeartMath e-book: *Using emWave® Technology For Children With ADHD - An Evidence-Based Intervention* by Jeff Goelitz Educational Specialist Institute of HeartMath and Dr. Tony Lloyd Chairman, ADHD Foundation, Liverpool, England.

emWave Desktop technology along with movement exercises, soothing music, and tapping. In order to have any effectiveness with the emWave, a child begins with basic breathing exercises. Often, the staff will have a child lie down on a massage table where he is better able to relax while practicing deep, rhythmic breathing. Once deep-breathing skills are established, then the child is ready for the other features of the emWave, including the games and Emotion Visualizer®. The results are very encouraging. Because parents want fast results (a minimum of eight weeks) in behavior regulation, the emWave plays a crucial role in teaching these children self-regulation skills." —**Madeline Falcone, MFT, director of the Falcone Institute, San Diego, Calif.**

Adult ADHD and Memory

An independent study conducted in the UK by Dr. Keith Wesnes with a group of thirty adults, concluded that learning and practicing the HeartMath coherence-building techniques appears to enhance the memory capacity of adults as well as improving self-reported calmness. Dr. Wesnes used the Cognitive Performance Testing Battery (CDR).

Cognitive Performance Testing Battery (CDR)
- Power of Attention
- Continuity of Attention
- Quality of Working Memory
- Quality of Episodic Secondary Memory
- Speed of Memory

The CDR assessed the ability to access memory, the quality of long term memory and short-term memory. Dr. Wesnes compared results from HeartMath practice to a placebo and to the best pharmaceutical memory-enhancing agent available.

The HeartMath results showed significant improvement in the quality of episodic (long-term) memory and a marginally significant improvement in the quality of working (short-term) memory. The observed gain of 12.6% in the quality of long-term memory was over a 7-week period during which coherence-building techniques were practiced. Dr. Wesnes reports the magnitude of improvement was significantly higher than the improvement in quality of memory obtained in a large clinical 14-week trial of the effects of a phyto-pharmaceutical memory enhancer (a gingko/ginseng combination) on the memory of healthy volunteers.

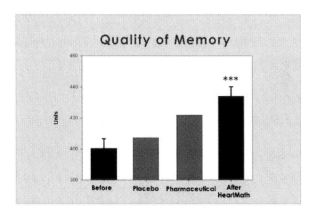

Effects of emWave Game-Based Training on Attention Problems in Anxious Children

Another study examined the effects of using with the emWave Desktop's games along with psycho-educational behavioral practices on 23 participants, ages 9 to 17, who were clinically diagnosed with anxiety disorders. The anxiety was strong enough in these children that they had ADHD-like symptoms. Anxiety and worry robbed these children of their capacity to pay full attention or concentrate on details in normal environments such as home or school. The average age of the children was 12.7 years. Twelve children were assigned to the intervention group, and the other 11 were placed on a waiting-list control group (those waiting to participate in an intervention after final measures are taken).

The Attention Problems Scale from the Child Behavior Checklist (CBCL) was used to measure pre- and post-results. Results showed significant differences in the post-test part of the Attention Problem Scale between the control group and intervention group. The parents also reported significant improvements in their children's attention compared to the waiting-list control group.

Test Scores and Coherence Baseline Increase

The U.S. Department of Education funded a large randomized controlled study carried out in collaboration with Claremont University's Graduate School of Education involving nearly 1000 tenth grade students from two large California high schools. The intention of the study was to see if HeartMath techniques and emWave training would reduce text anxiety and improve reading and math test scores. The grant was made based on smaller successful pilot studies including the following:

Dade County, Florida - Interpersonal Skills / Mental Attitude Improvement
In this study, after learning HeartMath techniques, students felt more motivated at school, were more focused in their school work and better able to organize and manage their time, both at school and at home. Their leadership and communication skills improved, and harmful behavior problems decreased. The children also felt more comfortable with themselves, were more assertive and independent in their decision making, more resistant to the demands of peer pressure and better able to manage their stress, anger and negative internal self-talk. In essence, the children showed increased satisfaction and control over their lives while with friends, at school and around their families. Notably, these significant improvements occurred within a short period of time. A follow up analysis indicated that many of these changes were sustained over the following six months. After observing the improvements in their children's attitudes, behavior and performance, many of the students' parents attended HeartMath trainings for themselves.

Minneapolis, Minnesota – Test Score Improvement
High school seniors who received a 3-week training in HeartMath learning enhancement skills demonstrated substantial improvements in test scores and passing rates on state-required math and reading tests. Students also experienced significant reductions in hostility, depression and other key indices of psychological distress after learning HeartMath tools.

Phoenix, Arizona – Reading Efficiency Improvement
Fourteen days of instruction in the HeartMath techniques allowed a special education class of fifth and sixth graders to significantly improve their reading proficiency.

"All 4th grades have completed the HeartMath program, and our parents are singing its praises. Parents report that kids are 'Freeze Framing' before dance or sporting performances, when fighting with a sibling and on and on! Our statewide writing scores came back, and once again we are #1 in the state (five years running). Through this program, our kids really take control of their emotions and channel things in a positive direction." **—Amanda Travis Simon, fourth-grade math/language arts teacher, Pine View School, Sarasota, Florida**

"Through the emWave Desktop, my students were able to identify what emotions interfered with their performance and then, using some of the HeartMath skills, neutralize those emotions so their brains could function better. Even the best students found it helpful." **—Gail Haase, director of development and research, Trinity Christian Schools, Las Vegas, NV**

The US Department of Education funded-study utilized a HeartMath program called TestEdge® along with the emWave Desktop. The results were a significant reduction in test anxiety as well as higher test scores. The post-intervention mean test score in tenth grade CST English-Language Arts was significantly higher for the intervention school—by a margin of approximately 10 points—than for the control school. Moreover, this improvement in test performance was associated with a significant reduction of test anxiety in the intervention school relative to the control school. When matched on baseline test scores, four groups of students, ranging from 50 to 129 in size, had significant increases in test performance (on average 10 to 25 points). Three of these groups had an increase in English test scores and the fourth group in Math test scores.

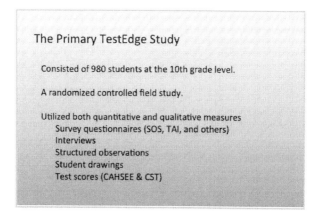

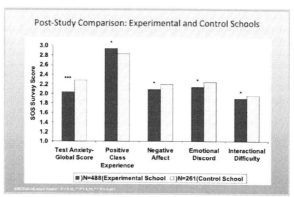

The study also measured a sub group of students resting state HRV to determine their level of HRV and how much natural HRV coherence each student had before and after they learned and practiced the self-regulation skills. The graph on page 70 shows a representative example of two students and the change in their resting HRV levels and natural coherence before and after the program was taught, about four months. The data suggests that when students self-manage their stress using coherence-building methods over a sustained time period it enabled them to increase their coherence baseline (the amount of coherence naturally occurring in their HRV) and achieve both a significant reduction in test-related anxiety and a corresponding improvement in standardized test scores—a real-world measure of cognitive performance.

"Over 70 percent of the participants surveyed felt the skills they had learned in the TestEdge program were of significant help on the MCAS (Massachusetts Comprehensive Assessment System tests) and all of them felt the program was of some aid. Nearly 90 percent of the participants believed that they performed better on the test using these techniques than they would have otherwise. MCAS Math scores showed a 16% average improvement."

—John Keppel, teacher, Stoughton High School, Stoughton, Mass.

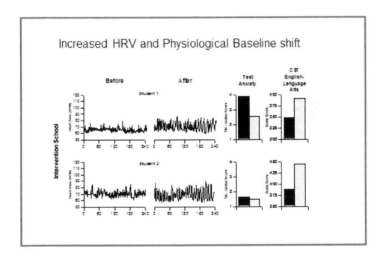

The coherence baseline shift can be seen in the before and after HRV traces in this graph. The coherence baseline shift in students correlated with improved self-regulation, reduced test anxiety (25% had been handicapped by test anxiety) and improved test scores.

U.S. Military

The U.S. Military have been employing heart coherence training in a HeartMath program, called The Coherence Advantage™, supported with emWave technology to improve resilience, cognitive performance, situational awareness and decision-making under high pressure. Cognitive function problems are one of hallmarks of PTSD in combat veterans. Many veteran's hospitals and clinics are using the HeartMath techniques and technology to help soldiers and veterans manage PTSD. One military study involved a brief HeartMath training including practice with the emWave over a few weeks. The results were improved memory, and learning, as well as the ability to encode the information. Most importantly, there was a significantly improved ability to self-regulate (ability to inhibit triggers and negative behaviors) which most likely facilitated the other results.

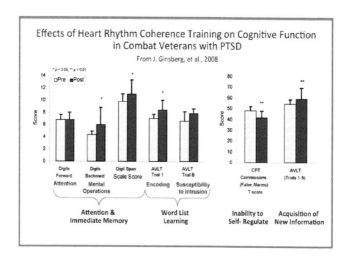

This graph shows improvements in various cognitive function measures prior to and after training and four weeks practice with HeartMath techniques and emWave technology to increase heart coherence. The results also found that increases in coherence were predictive of improvements in commissions (the ability to self-regulate) and the ability to absorb new information.

TBI – Traumatic Brain Injury

Brain injuries cause impairments that affect physical, cognitive and psychosocial functioning in people of any age. Usually, deficits in executive functioning present more obstacles to a person's full return from TBI than physical or medical complications do. Fundamental to executive functioning is self-regulation, the ability to inhibit impulses, exercise restraint, adapt as needed and turn passive experience into productive activity.

A significant deficit in self-regulation is a hallmark of individuals with brain injury. Studies show that self-regulation training that incorporates HRV coherence feedback can improve regulation of emotions and behavior; and, in turn, improve cognitive functioning in individuals with moderate-to-severe chronic brain injury. HRV coherence is associated with improving executive functions—attention, flexibility of thought and self-directed control of emotions and behaviors. A study on heart rate variability biofeedback, executive functioning and chronic brain injury published in *Brain Injury*, February 2013, found that individuals with severe and chronic brain injury demonstrated improvements in HRV coherence levels after a relatively short period of time. Even individuals with severe neurological damage were able to modify their HRV coherence.

An example is Jasmina Agrillo's story of recovery. *"Never in my wildest imaginings did I ever think I would go on this journey! It just wasn't in my life plan. On March 5, 2001, I was operated on for the removal of a very large brain tumor. About a year before finally collapsing at home from an undiagnosed brain tumor I had begun experiencing myself physically, emotionally and mentally as "falling apart." My symptoms included terrible headaches that were causing visual disturbances, coordination and balance problems, mood swings and irrational thinking and behavior. During the next year my symptoms worsened as I visited several doctors who failed to diagnose the source of my debilitating symptoms. Finally one day I was unable to walk and began losing some vision. At the Emergency Room an attending physician ordered a CT scan. I then met my neurosurgeon who informed me that I had a very large frontal lobe bi-lateral* meningioma brain tumor and I was immediately transferred to Maine Medical Center to prepare for emergency surgery within a few days. After studying the results of my MRI and cerebral angiogram my neurosurgeon informed me that the tumor was slightly bigger than a lemon and intersected a main artery in 3 locations. The surgery could be long and complicated. As I was facing the possibility of my own death, I was also thinking "what's it going to be like if I live? Isn't brain intelligence everything, what we rely on, what we know?" I prayed that I be allowed to live, to get a second chance for a whole new life!

The surgery was very successful. However, nothing could have prepared me for the debilitation of brain recovery. I faced many physical and cognitive challenges. In the physical I had coordination/balance problems that were further complicated by seizures. In acute recovery there was the constant pain as the ear to ear incision and neural tissue healed, drug side effects, dizziness, sleeplessness and fatigue to cope with. Attention deficit, short -term memory loss, speech and language difficulties and impulse control were my cognitive challenges. I was also deeply, traumatized by the fear, uncertainty and suffering from not being diagnosed for a year and the adult baby I found myself to be after surgery. And just like a baby I needed to be nourished by love and care from others. I am not able to convey to you the full devastating impact this had on my family.

At ten months into recovery, I seemed to have reached a plateau in my cognitive recovery and was thinking that my brain had healed as much as it could. It was then that I began practicing the HeartMath System. I learned to use techniques that combine heart focus, breath and positive emotion to create a balanced physiology that is referred to as 'coherence'. With a tool called Quick Coherence® I was able to feel good in the moment, a state I could achieve anytime and place. It was almost like a magic pill! This was especially appealing to me because it was easy to do and non drug related.

By learning to send feelings that create coherence into my body while breathing through my heart, I was able to gain more control of my physiology than I ever had before. To help me do this I used the emWave Desktop that allowed me to see in real time the changing rhythms of my heart. I learned to produce more smooth and coherent (balanced) heart rhythms which signaled all parts of my brain and nervous system to operate in sync. This had a tremendous impact on how my brain functioned. The effects were immediate. I felt more peaceful, calm, focused and clear thinking—no small thing in brain injury recovery!

Regular practice of sustaining heart coherence helped me to maintain a balance in my physiology over a longer period of time. This helped stabilize my brain, enabling it to heal faster while I stayed more mentally and emotionally balanced. I even gained pain control. Over time, under the guidance of my neurologist, I was able to wean off seizure medications and pain meds for migraines.

The first month into my heart tools practice I noticed cognitive improvement in my ability to stay focused and to remember incoming information. By learning to intentionally focus on a positive heart feeling such as care, love, compassion and appreciation I was able to gain a, healthy, balanced, caring perspective and to act on it. After seeing how amazingly well I was recovering my neurosurgeon commented. "Do you know how lucky you are to be having this recovery?" My cognitive recovery has been most profound and successful. It has been exciting and like a miracle to experience the re-wiring of my neural circuitry – almost like I grew another brain! I have re-gained full use of all my cognitive functions. I have a new normal now.

Jasmina, now a HeartMath coach, teaches HeartMath to other brain injury survivors. Here are a few of their stories:

Tom-"Tom's brain injury recovery goals were to use heart coherence tools to help relieve anxiety, to help his attention, memory and reading comprehension, and have more clarity in making decisions. I began teaching him Neutral, the first two steps of the Quick Coherence technique. He was able to make the heart-brain connection, noticing that he felt less anxiety and stress in his body, felt calmer and able to think more clearly. He liked the feeling of being in a calm neutral feeling place. It gave him a feeling of having more control when so much of his brain injury deficits were beyond his control. Tom was excited to go home and look up the word Neutral in the dictionary.

To help his brain retain the steps of the Quick Coherence technique he needed to say it, write it and read it in his notebook which he carries with him at all times. Tom reported on his second session that he practices getting Neutral a lot during the day and its becoming a habit. His anxiety is better, he feels calmer and he's sleeping better. His notebook and cue cards were very helpful to remind him to practice—he posted them around his apartment. At our fourth session Tom indicated that he was ready to practice getting coherent on the emWave PC! It was a challenge for him because of his attention deficit issues to look at the HRV pattern and get coherent. Considering all the challenges he was able to get 20% high coherence in less than 5 minutes!

Tom's embarrassed feelings about being judged for his brain injury deficits often prevented him from communicating with others and getting the help and information he needs. He often misses going on favorite outings because of this. He was very excited to tell me that this time he recognized his embarrassed feeling, moved through it by getting neutral and was able to make the call to get information about a special outing. Recognizing this shift gave him the confidence to do it again when the embarrassing feeling came up. He became so successful that he was able to advocate for himself and get the speech and language rehabilitation he very much needed.

By Tom's seventh session, he was able to maintain coherence on the emWave Balloon Game while listening to the music, an indication that his multi-tasking attention deficit issues were improving! Gaining more control of his attention issues seemed to be the gateway to using coherence to help improve his memory. In subsequent sessions Tom would practice sustaining coherence hooked up to the emWave PC while playing memory games with a deck of cards. Appreciating himself and *his accomplishments became part of his daily coherence practice. His ability to think more clearly and make decisions was getting better. He felt confident enough to consider vocational rehabilitation."*

Sally- *"I met Sally at a Brain Injury support group presentation in a rehabilitation facility. She was 4 plus years into recovery and volunteered for the group to experience the emWave Desktop. Sally's brain injury happened in the summer of 1999 as a result of a car accident. She was injured in her left temporal lobe, which is the area of the brain that processes memory, hearing, understanding language, organization and sequencing. This was a mild, closed head injury that didn't show visible signs in MRI testing at the hospital. She was therefore released not knowing she had a brain injury. Her main brain injury symptoms were: fatigue, attention deficit, planning/ organization, problem solving and anxiety about her condition. She also had sensorimotor impairments as seizures, sound and light sensitivity, dizziness and balance problems. After several months of not being able to function very well in her life and work, she sought rehabilitation and learned in her neurological evaluation that she had a brain injury.*

After the 15 minute heart coherence training session, Sally was very fatigued and needed a cool down rest period to move into a quiet deeper relaxation response. This recovery rest period took about 35 minutes before she was able to drive home. Normally, recovery from a seizure episode would take hours of lying on the couch with her earplugs in. Before leaving my office she said, "This is powerful stuff!"

Mark-*"On a cold, rainy, December night, Mark, a police officer, experienced a brain injury as a result of his work. He lost consciousness for a brief period of time and had post traumatic amnesia for less than 24 hours. His persistent post concussion symptoms included: headache, dizziness, sleep disturbance, irritability, changes in personality, memory problems, depression, difficulty in problem solving and diminished attention span. The mild brain injury he sustained was a life altering event—he could no longer serve as a police officer in his pre-injury capacity. The insurance company* was eager to get him rehabilitated and so the emWave Desktop and my sessions were fully covered as stress management feedback techniques. At our very first session Mark was able to practice getting coherent on the emWave without difficulty, which he purchased to begin practicing at home. Here is what Mark has to say in an interview with me about how HeartMath techniques have helped him in recovery:

> 'HeartMath has helped me control my stress and control pain. My TBI was a very stressful and life altering event. HeartMath allowed me to feel positive emotions. Using the HeartMath techniques I am able to be more attentive for longer periods of time. I have the ability to remember many more things than I had before. It has helped me through many projects that I would have otherwise not been able to accomplish. I have the ability to control my emotions much more than I was before HeartMath. Although I still struggle from time to time with depression, I have the tools with HeartMath to diminish the length of episodes. I am a more peaceful man; my family has really seen a difference.'

"I have been using the emWave2® handheld with soldiers returning from combat and have been more than pleased with results. The emWave surpasses all of my expectations, as it is very sensitive, and because of that has proven useful in resource building of safe place/calm place mental relaxation, and to ensure that my clients are emotionally congruent with their words and able to leave sessions more relaxed.

"It is so sensitive that I was taking a client through safe place/calm place after some desensitization work and he was relaxed and 'green' until I mentioned the lake he has in his calm place. I asked him about the lake after the emWave turned red. He reported that he cannot swim. The sensitivity of the emWave picked up on this and he decided to omit the lake from his relaxing mental imagery and get back to a relaxed state. Thanks for a great tool! It has become an essential part of therapy with the soldiers."

—**Travis Slonecker, LCWS, Fort Knox, Ky**

"Mark has also been using Quick Coherence to help him stay focused and clear to solve math problems in taking tests as part of his vocational rehabilitation. "I believe HeartMath has allowed my doctors to discontinue many medications. I went from six medicines down to two since I have been using HeartMath."

What More People Are Saying about HeartMath and Brain Fitness

"I have used various curricula and insight therapy techniques with my DIS (designated instructional services) groups for high school students with anger management, ADHD, substance abuse, test anxiety and other issues. By far, the most effective program I have found for addressing these issues is HeartMath." **—Sam Bouman, MS, PPS, school psychologist, Glendora School District, California**

"I managed inpatient and outpatient PTSD programs at a VA facility for over 20 years and used HeartMath since the very early days. Every returning war-zone vet should have the opportunity to rewire their nervous system. I have done this with hundreds of heavy combat military personnel and most can learn to do this in 3–4 weeks. I am very big on HRV feedback and highly recommend HeartMath products." **—ARMY CLINICAL PSYCHOLOGIST**

"I used the emWave to calm myself down before my exams. The results were staggering. I received 84%, and 85% respectively on my statistics and forensic exams. Now I know how to calm myself down before and during an exam." **—Shannon Kimmitt, student, University of British Columbia, Okanagan**

"What impressed me as I watched the students was the quality of questions they were asking as they worked together on a math puzzle. They looked at the problem from different perspectives and came up with an answer but it was wrong. They revised their thinking and found a better solution. These are the skills they'll need for work in the 21st century." **—Rami Meuth, district director of curriculum TestEdge® National Demonstration Study**

"I use HeartMath a lot! When my kids are out of sorts, they go to the emWave Desktop center. All of them are able to quiet themselves and get focused."
—Kim Wise, third-grade teacher, Justina Road Elementary, Jacksonville, Fla.

*"Through the emWave Desktop, my students were able to identify what emotions interfered with their performance and then, using some of the HeartMath skills, neutralize those emotions so their brains could function better. Even the best students found it helpful."***—Gail Haase, director of development and research, Trinity Christian Schools, Las Vegas, NV**

"I will hook a child up to the emWave Desktop technology and assess their current status in terms of heart-rate-variability patterns and coherence ratios. This is the beginning baseline. Then I immediately instruct them in the Quick Coherence Technique with a big emphasis on breathing. To jump-start the breathing practice, I have the child place his or her hand on the chest and feel the breath coming in and then going out. Five seconds on the in-breath and five seconds on the out-breath. They feel the breath with the hand. It becomes a kinesthetic experience. Meanwhile, I am paying attention to the amplitude of the heart-rhythm wave on the computer screen. Bigger waves mean deeper breaths and more oxygen being distributed into a child's brain, more autonomic nervous-system balance and the stoppage of cortisol production. After a short while, a child becomes noticeably calmer and quieter. I point out the difference between their current state and the state they had when they first came in. Each session on the emWave lasts between three and eight minutes. Normally, it will take five sessions before I think they are ready to advance to the software games. This criteria is based on a child's ability to calm down as indicated by body language, but also from the visual evidence of the taller wave forms (in the heart-rate-variability pattern).They enjoy playing the games very much. Making the balloon go higher, adding coins to their bank account (Rainbow Game) or coloring a garden adds fun to the learning experience. If I work with a child for four to six months, there is a good chance we will see positive benefits both at home and at school." **—Dee Edmonson, RN, director of the Neurotherapy Center of Plano, TX**

"Typically I introduce the emWave Desktop as a primary intervention to assist students in developing the self-management skills needed to cope with stress. I find it very useful because it offers visual feedback. Students see the results of their actions. And it is so easy to use."—**Vern Russell, director of Student Counseling Services, Auburn University, Auburn, Ala.**

"About 320 students are introduced to the emWave as part of my cooperative learning and leadership program each year. We explore what emotion is and how emotions can help or hinder what we do. We get into "what is coherence" and how that helps the mind and body perform better, like with test-taking. They all get it. They even tell me to use it when I get upset." —**Linda Gancitano, health teacher, Driftwood Middle Academy of Health and Wellness, Hollywood, Florida**

"At a time of increased emphasis on student performance as measured by various standardized tests, the HeartMath TestEdge program can make an enormous difference in helping students perform up to their potential." —**Lourdes Arguelles, Ph.D. Professor of Education, Claremont Graduate University**

"We have had great success using HeartMath's TestEdge Program with thousands of our students in middle and high school and we are very excited about being able to give our elementary students the same advantage." —**Kathy Reutman Bryant, executive director, student services, Boone County Schools, Kentucky**

"In the 40 years I have worked in this field, I have found HeartMath Interventions to be the most effective methods for transforming stress and emotional turmoil into well-being."—**Tom McDermott, NCC, LMHC, director of counseling services, Niagara University, New York**

"Using the emWave Personal Stress Reliever has enabled me to recognize the effects of stress on my body at any given time, which then allows me to use the HeartMath techniques to immediately help relieve this stress

position. My recent tournament performances in Germany and Holland were helped by the use of HeartMath. The emWave can recognize stress levels not otherwise detectable." **—Ian Woosnam, United Kingdon, 2006 European Ryder Cup captain and 1991 Masters winner**

"The December test scores showed a 16% improvement in math scores and a number of very positive comments from students ... in the pilot study." **—Prudence Goodale, assistant superintendent, Stoughton Public Schools, Mass.**

"The detailed information presented in this report ... provides impressive evidence of the effectiveness of the TestEdge program. For students who were trained to use the TestEdge program to manage their stress, this resulted in significant reductions in the Test Anxiety Inventory scores and corresponding improvement in scores on standard measures of academic performance."
—Charles D. Spielberger, Ph.D., ABPP, psychologist; author – State-Trait Anxiety Inventory, and Test Anxiety Inventory; distinguished research professor of psychology and director, University of South Florida

"I have PTSD and have had nightmares almost every night all my life. The first time I used emWave right before sleep, I had my first night's sleep with NO nightmares, and it still works every night! Also, having once been very articulate, I was very frustrated by memory problems affecting word recall. I struggled to find even simple every day words as I stammered, felt stupid and was often unable to express what I wanted. A few days after using emWave daily, I actually found myself discussing some fairly deep, abstract subjects fluently and effortlessly with NO word recall problem! It's also helped me with anxiety – it helps me calm before difficult tasks, calm after upsets and get clearer to make important decisions. emWave has improved my life in many ways!"

—Becky F., Psychiatric Social Worker

Your Brain Fitness Companion: emWave® or Inner Balance™

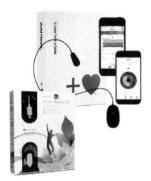

HeartMath's Heart Rate Variability (HRV) technology is a scientifically validated system that trains you into an optimal high performance state in which the heart, brain and nervous system are operating in sync and in balance. We call this state coherence. HeartMath's HRV products measure your coherence level, store your data and connect you to the HeartCloud™ for community support and rewards. As you increase your coherence level, your ability to focus and take charge of emotional reactions improves and you have greater access to your heart's intuitive guidance system for making effective choices.

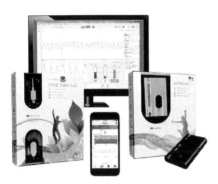

The emWave2® or Inner Balance™
Portable and convenient ways to reduce stress, balance your emotions, increase your cognitive functions and enhance performance. Used just a few minutes a day, this simple-to-use technology helps to transform anger, anxiety or frustration into inner peace, ease and mental clarity. Health, communication and relationships improve.

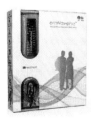

emWave Pro for PC & Mac
Using a pulse sensor plugged into a USB port, emWave Pro collects and translates HRV (heart rate variability) coherence data into user-friendly graphics. It provides a Coherence Coach®, fun visualizers and games that respond to your coherence level. emWave Pro and emWave Pro Plus are multi-user and ideal for classrooms and for health professionals to keep track of client data and progress.

www.heartmath.com or call 1–800–450–9111

Training and Certification Programs

Add Heart Daily Calls
Dial in or log in to join a 10 minute call with a HeartMath staff trainer to increase your mental and emotional fitness and practice the Heart Lock-In® Technique together.

Become an Add Heart Facilitator
Become an approved facilitator to learn and share with others some of the science that underpins the HeartMath system, an effective three-step technique for getting into coherence, and how to use the Inner Balance Trainer. In this online course, you learn how to share what you are learning in personal and professional situations.

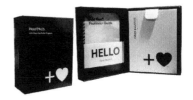

Become a HeartMath® Certified Coach/Mentor
Learn via an 8 week telephone course HeartMath's scientifically–validated tool set and how to teach these tools to clients. HeartMath Coach/Mentors are licensed to teach the HeartMath System in a one-on-one setting.

Become a HeartMath® Certified Trainer
Attend a full immersion 4.5 day certification program. HeartMath Certified Trainers are licensed to provide HeartMath workshops in a 6 hour program, and in shorter modules, or to embed HeartMath modules, techniques, tools and scientific concepts into other training programs.

Become a Licensed HeartMath® Health Professional
The HeartMath Interventions Certification Program includes 6 one hour interactive webinars and video presentations. Health professionals learn how to use HeartMath techniques and technology with patients in various therapeutic and clinical applications.

HeartMath Institute

HeartMath Institute (HMI) is nonprofit organization that researches and develops scientifically based tools to help people bridge the connection between their hearts and minds. It also provides HeartMath programs to social service agencies, and curricula for children and schools pre K-college. **www.heartmath.org.**

Call 1–800-450–9111 or visit www.heartmath.com

Heart Intelligence, Connecting with the Intuitive Guidance of the Heart

By Doc Childre, Howard Martin, Deborah Rozman Ph.D. and Rollin McCraty Ph.D.

Our newest book, Heart Intelligence, provides breakthrough research linking the physical heart to the spiritual (energetic) heart. This book provides simple techniques for accessing our heart's intuitive intelligence for moment–to–moment guidance and discernment

Transforming Depression: The HeartMath® Solution to Feeling Overwhelmed, Sad, and Stressed
by Doc Childre and Deborah Rozman, Ph.D.

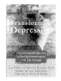

Transforming Anxiety: The HeartMath Solution for Overcoming Fear and Worry and Creating Serenity
by Doc Childre and Deborah Rozman, Ph.D.

Transforming Stress: The HeartMath Solution For Relieving Worry, Fatigue, and Tension
by Doc Childre and Deborah Rozman, Ph.D.

Transforming Anger, The HeartMath Solution for Letting Go of Rage, Frustration and Irritation
by Doc Childre and Deborah Rozman, Ph.D.

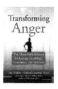

The HeartMath Solution
by Doc Childre and Howard Martin

www.heartmath.com or call 1–800–450–9111